Pioneering Health in London, 1935–2000

The Peckham Experiment, conducted between 1935 and 1950 in the London Pioneer Health Centre, was one of the most talked-about social experiments of the twentieth century. Families from the South London neighbourhood of Peckham were invited to use the facilities of a radiantly modern building. They were encouraged to freely choose and organize their leisure activities, taking advantage of a swimming pool, a gymnasium, and a self-service cafeteria. In doing so, both their health status and interaction with other members of the nascent centre-community were closely observed by a team of physicians.

The first research monograph on the history of the experiment building on archival sources, this book combines a micro-historical perspective with methods from the history of science. It shows how bio-medical holism and evolutionary theories typical of the interwar years informed research on social life in the centre. But it also reveals that the "guinea pigs", too, were trying to make sense of the research they were taking part in. The outcome was an ambiguous social laboratory that generated new insights into the power of social groups to self-organize, which were soon discussed all over the world – and continue to haunt British political debates today.

David Kuchenbuch is Assistant Professor in the Department of History at Justus-Liebig-University Giessen, Germany.

Routledge Studies in the History of Science, Technology and Medicine

For the full list of titles in the series, please visit: https://www.routledge.com/Routledge-Studies-in-the-History-of-Science-Technology-and-Medicine/book-series/HISTSCI

Pioneering Health in London, 1935–2000

The Peckham Experiment

David Kuchenbuch

Translated by Alex Skinner

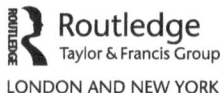
Routledge
Taylor & Francis Group

LONDON AND NEW YORK

Originally published as *Das Peckham-Experiment – Eine Mikro- und Wissensgeschichte des Londoner "Pioneer Health Centre" im 20. Jahrhundert* by Böhlau-Verlag, copyright 2014. Translated from German by permission of Böhlau-Verlag.

English translation first published 2019
by Routledge
2 Park Square, Milton Park, Abingdon, Oxon OX14 4RN

and by Routledge
52 Vanderbilt Avenue, New York, NY 10017

First issued in paperback 2020

Routledge is an imprint of the Taylor & Francis Group, an informa business

© 2019 David Kuchenbuch

British Library Cataloguing in Publication Data
A catalogue record for this book is available from the British Library

Library of Congress Cataloging in Publication Data
A catalog record for this book has been requested

ISBN 13: 978-0-36-758457-3 (pbk)
ISBN 13: 978-1-138-72291-0 (hbk)

Typeset in Times New Roman
by Taylor & Francis Books

The Translation of this work was funded by Geisteswissenschaften International – Translation Funding for Humanities and Social Sciences from Germany, a joint initiative of the Fritz Thyssen Foundation, the German Federal Foreign Office, the collecting society VG WORT and the Börsenverein des Deutschen Buchhandels (German Publishers & Booksellers Association).

Contents

vi *Contents*

Figures

Acknowledgments

Anyone writing a case study based on original sources will incur a tremendous debt of gratitude to archivists. In my case this means, above all, the staff of the Wellcome Library in London, but also the National Archives in Kew, the London Metropolitan Archives and the Southwark Local History Archives, to all of whom I am deeply grateful. My thanks also go to the Deutsche Forschungsgemeinschaft (DFG), whose financial support facilitated the research, writing and printing of the 2014 German-language version of this book, along with the History Department at the Justus-Liebig-Universität Gießen, which provided me with the necessary infrastructure. On a personal level I would particularly like to thank Friedrich Lenger, not least for suggesting that I follow the money trail that enabled me to make a reality of the present book, and Ingrun Berg, who ensured that the administration of the DFG project in Gießen was so headache-free.

That my findings are now available in an updated and slightly revised English-language edition is thanks to the "Geisteswissenschaften International" programme, through which the Fritz Thyssen Foundation, VG Wort, The German Publishers and Booksellers Association (Börsenverein des Deutschen Buchhandels) and the German Federal Foreign Office support the translation of texts in the social sciences and humanities. But I would never have obtained this funding if not for the support of the Böhlau-Verlag publishing house – particularly Dorothee Rheker-Wunsch, whose professional supervision was such a boon to the first edition – and Rob Langham at Taylor & Francis who, despite a number of delays, enthusiastically expedited a publication project rather unusual for a British publisher. The Pioneer Health Foundation (PHF) and the Sir Halley Stewart Trust kindly gave permission to publish numerous images and quotations. Finally, Alex Skinner has produced a judicious translation into English.

The content of the book, too, owes much to the efforts and ideas of many individuals. Friedrich Lenger and Willibald Steinmetz read the manuscript of the German edition and supported its inclusion in Böhlau's "Industrial World" series. Earlier I had the privilege of presenting and discussing the project's design at a number of graduate seminars, colloquia and workshops: in Munich, Utrecht, Glasgow, Bielefeld, in Gießen on several occasions and in Havixbeck near Münster. My sincere thanks to the participants and initiators of these discussions. Comments from Maria Daldrup, Martin Kindtner, Helmut Lethen and Dirk Thomaschke helped me sharpen up my ideas. Gregor Harbusch gave me tips on sources and made my research in Zürich a delight. I also want to thank Elena Meilicke for putting me in touch with Nikolaus Perneczky, and the latter for facilitating contact with the residents of the Pioneer Centre. My sincere thanks to Simon Leary for welcoming me into his home, to Emily Charkin for sending me her master's thesis on "Peckham", and to Lisa Curtice of the PHF, who was not only very supportive in the process of obtaining printing permissions but also pointed me to interesting projects that fathom the potential of "Peckham" today. Last but not least I am grateful to the critical readers of the various versions of this book: Hanna Engelmeier, Ylva Eriksson-Kuchenbuch, Thomas Etzemüller, Till Greite, Ludolf Kuchenbuch, Timo Luks, Sabrina Röstel-Kuchenbuch and Anette Schlimm.

Berlin, May 2018

Abbreviations

AA	Architectural Association School of Architecture
BMA	British Medical Association
CIAM	Congrès Internationaux d'Architecture Moderne
COS	Charity Organisation Society
GLC	Greater London Council
GP	general practitioner
LCC	London County Council
LLP	London Labour Party
LSE	London School of Economics and Political Science
MP	member of Parliament
MRC	Medical Research Council
NHS	National Health Service
PEP	Political and Economic Planning
PHC	Pioneer Health Centre, Peckham
RAF	Royal Air Force
RIBA	Royal Institute of British Architects
SMA	Socialist Medical Association
UN	United Nations
UNESCO	United Nations Educational, Scientific and Cultural Organization
WHO	World Health Organization

1 Introduction

The Peckham Experiment, so the story goes, was a treasure-trove of valuable insights. In 1926 the small Pioneer Health Centre (PHC) opened on Queen's Road in Peckham, a working-class district of South London. Here physician couple George Scott Williamson (1884–1953) and Innes Hope Pearse (1889–1978) tested out a form of health care centred on the informal impartation of basic knowledge about hygiene and preventative practices. The centre was conceived as a kind of leisure club – there was a club room, cards and board games, and the directors even applied for a licence to sell tobacco and beer – as this promised to lure in the local residents. On site, through personal contact, they would then be taught one thing above all else: responsibility for their own bodies and families. The doctors were also interested in the compensatory effects of the social environment on medical conditions, devoting themselves to what modern-day social medicine considers situational prevention, in contrast to behavioural prevention.

The success of this pilot project (which came to an end in 1929) encouraged its initiators to plan a new, significantly larger centre just a few streets away, on St Mary's Road. This was inaugurated in 1935 and remained open until the outbreak of the Second World War, before resuming its work in 1946 for another four years. In addition to the doctors' examination rooms, the building that housed the centre, designed by architect-engineer Sir William Owen – which quickly became a modernist icon in the UK – had a swimming pool, a gymnasium, club rooms, a library, a nursery and a self-service cafeteria. It was intended to serve up to 2,000 families. The residents of Peckham were offered unlimited use of the centre's facilities for a comparatively small fee – on two conditions. It was only open to families, rather than individuals, living in the centre's immediate vicinity. Upon admission and once a year these families had to submit to a medical examination, in which the physician not only assessed the health of individual family members but discussed it with the entire family in a so-called family consultation. Otherwise the doctors' work was limited to observing those using the centre and providing medical advice upon request. No attempt was made to organize activities. There were no courses, fixed schedules or age restrictions. It was left entirely up to centre members to decide when and how to make use of the facilities provided – which included sporting equipment, musical instruments, tools and children's toys.

The doctors soon noticed some astonishing developments at the centre. First, after a brief chaotic phase the users themselves achieved a form of harmonious coexistence. Second, they began to show an interest in both their health and their fellows. This led to a reduction in illness but also to a generally happier, open atmosphere. So for the centre's directors (who subsequently published several books about it[1] that sparked off a lively international debate), the experiment's results were many-layered. Users had made the centre their own without outside interference and this – to cite the main thrust of these publications – had prompted them to willingly take responsibility for themselves and others, which had in turn bolstered the efficacy of medical advice. But according to the physicians – who had now begun to refer to themselves as biologists – the centre had not just brought about a measurable improvement in users' resistance to illness. It had also engendered more spontaneous, informal relations between them while simultaneously making them more willing to work on themselves. In other words, it had unleashed their creative interest in their own potential. Rather than coercion or instruction, planning or propaganda, or even classical paternalistic charity, what had helped users achieve a healthy existence – and for the researchers this always meant an active, autonomous and integrated one – was an environment replete with appealing activities, social stimulation and freely circulating knowledge.

A medical pilot scheme had thus turned into a research project that seemed to confirm a downright anthropological thesis. But it happened at the wrong time politically. Much to its users' disappointment the centre had to close in 1950. Its directors' unconventional approach, its focus on nuclear families and the tremendous freedoms the latter enjoyed within it clashed with the administrative structure and expertocratic character of the new British welfare system. It was particularly out of sync with the National Health Service (NHS), which had been introduced two years earlier, above all because of its focus on curative functions, specifically treatment in hospitals. Pearse and Scott Williamson, however, were unwilling to accept changes in the experimental conditions, which they feared might gravely disrupt the process of self-organization observed among users. Every attempt to found a new centre was scuppered by the dirigist zeitgeist.

A laboratory of the present?

Like a spectral presence, this portrayal has continued to inform a great deal of historical research on the centre ever since, as well as the non-scientific accounts, a prominent example being the BBC documentary *Health before the NHS: The Road to Recovery*, broadcast in January 2016.[2] Since the 1950s "Peckham" has been rediscovered on several occasions. At times it has served researchers as they have looked back to the future from a normative perspective, while at others it has functioned as a model for historically based analyses of the modern world. For example, in 1966 British anarchist Colin Ward devoted an entire special issue of the journal *Anarchy* to the centre. For him and his colleagues it was a "laboratory of anarchism". It had, Ward believed, furnished scientific proof that what he regarded as a functioning social order would emerge of its own accord in the absence of authority or top-down expertise. The Peckham Experiment, he concluded, was an "exemplary parable […], of the way things ought to be done", particularly against the background of the post-war welfare state with its bureaucracies and hierarchies.[3] While projects of this kind were limited to a niche environment in the planning-obsessed 1960s, they attracted greater interest in the institution-sceptical climate of subsequent decades. Time and again the centre now drew praise as an alternative to an expensive and allegedly inefficient NHS that deprived users of their voice, as for example in an essay entitled "Total Participation, Total Health: Reinventing the Peckham Health Centre for the 1990's".[4] As recently as 2007 *Guardian* columnist Jonathan Freedland suggested that the then Labour government ought to take a look at the centre as it attempted to reform the welfare state. For him it could point to a middle way between the social policy approaches of various British prime ministers, namely the "uber-Blairite worship of choice and marketisation" on the one hand and the "Brownite desire to get a grip [by] submitting every ward to a 'deep clean'" on the other.[5] In fact, according to Freedland the powerful "Whitehall state" had rushed the introduction of the NHS, nipping local self-management in the bud. It would, however, be a mistake to demonize post-war centralism as David Cameron was allegedly doing with his "self-described 'big idea' of social responsibility".[6]

Freedland's plea triggered a nuanced debate among readers of the newspaper's website. Commentators recalled anarchist and left-wing libertarian British traditions; they discussed the pros and cons of increased competition in the welfare state and of a demand-driven form of health care; and they argued about the tasks for which voluntary organizations ought to be responsible, whether these bodies be of a philanthropic, communitarian or cooperative nature.[7] It may come as little surprise that an interwar reform project should crop up in a later debate on the future of society. We need only think of the role played by the New Deal at least in the early days of the debate on Barack Obama's Patient Protection and Affordable Care Act. What is odd is that statements made in the context of the Peckham Experiment – as quoted by Freedland – seem so relevant to the present day. It was in fact the terms associated with the notion of *empowerment*, such as activity, participation, flexibility and creativity, that enabled a local social project of the 1930s to fuel a debate ultimately revolving around British society in the post-Thatcher era.[8]

From a critical perspective, this debate might prompt us to conclude that "Peckham" has detached itself entirely from historical time. Are activity, adaptability, creativity and a desire to network not key desiderata within flexible capitalism, whose core norm is the individual willingness to work on oneself? As many social scientists have pointed out, over the last few decades the welfare state has begun to focus less on redistributing wealth than on mobilizing people, often with the help of intermediary private welfare organizations.[9] This is bound up with an idea of society ever less informed by assumptions about its social and economic stratification. Instead it is underpinned by a "neosocial" distinction between citizens according to degrees of activity, a notion whose growing importance has been highlighted by German sociologist Stephan Lessenich.[10] In the mid 1960s Colin Ward perceived the Peckham Experiment as a laboratory of anarchism. Was it in fact an early testing ground for "modern-day governmentality", a Foucauldian attempt to encourage work on the self?[11]

This would appear to be the case if we turn to recent publications on the Pioneer Health Centre by architectural historians. They have described the Peckham Experiment as a novel regime of activation in miniature,[12] not infrequently by extrapolating from the centre's flexible ground plan to the social processes occurring within it. They assert that the unusually open construction, much of it divided only by glass partitions, facilitated circulation, mutual observation and spontaneous contact among users, prompting them to engage in activities.

This conclusion is often buttressed by comparisons with the other interwar London health centre of national renown: the Finsbury Health Centre. Opened in 1938, this was located to the north of the City and set up by the London County Council (LCC), dominated by the Labour Party from 1934 onwards.[13] The two institutions undoubtedly differed in many respects, despite starting out with similar motives – rooted in social medicine – and a similar modernist appearance. A more didactic and hierarchical space than "Peckham", "Finsbury" had been consciously established in a poorer district. Murals by T. Gordon Cullen in the entrance hall featured slogans propagating a hygienic lifestyle. The centre's highly differentiated ground plan, meanwhile, drew a clear boundary between medical staff and patients. The building, constructed by the Tecton group associated with Russian constructivist Berthold Lubetkin (which presented itself to the world as a team of no-nonsense technicians), featured clearly separated waiting rooms, reception areas and consulting rooms. It even had separate entrances for users, staff and deliveries. Extrapolating from these architectural differences, researchers have tended to view the two centres as representative of the competing social policy actors and approaches observable in the UK in the 1930s, prior to the establishment of the post-war welfare state. On the one hand we have a socialist local government, on the other, a philanthropically inclined private initiative that some researchers perceive as socially conservative; in Peckham we see the principles of empowerment, participation and personal responsibility, but also a focus on the families, while Finsbury is characterized by the power of experts, redistribution and universal access to welfare benefits. In addition, the Finsbury Health Centre was designed to be a "megaphone for health" that would resound across a wide area, whereas the PHC was to function more subtly as a "magnet", pulling people in before subjecting them to its stimuli.[14]

The centre in the north of the city, it appears, was more successful over the medium term. At least, the stylized image of the building appears time and again in mid-twentieth-century Britain, displayed on a wartime poster under the heading "Your Britain, Fight For It Now" (and contrasted with a dilapidated slum building). Though in reality it was a city institution, the Finsbury Health Centre embodied the national government's sociopolitical promises within the context of the "people's war". From a history-of-mentality perspective, scholars have often viewed these promises as the foundation for the expansion of the welfare state after 1945. In contrast, it was not until the beginning of the end of the "classical" welfare state in the late 1970s that the Peckham Experiment began to make waves.

If we endorse this assessment, we might go even further and assert that "Peckham" did more than generate new, activating techniques of governance. In terms of the history of science (and to a certain extent the typology of historical eras) there is a great temptation to comprehend the centre in South London as a laboratory of post-modernity, yet one operating during the core phase of so-called high modernity, often characterized by historians as an era of social-technological interventionism.[15] In fact the present book is the by-product of a research project on modern social engineering, in other words, attempts by bourgeois social experts to "order" society. Certainly, in the post-war era even these social engineers – in my case German and Swedish city planners – abandoned the idea of the rigid planning of social structures, embraced citizen participation and even welcomed a certain degree of social dynamism.[16] Nonetheless, I was struck by the impartiality with which experts associated with the Peckham Experiment were already observing how people organized themselves in the 1930s – people that many of these experts' colleagues regarded as members of a disquieting social stratum in desperate need of education. I wanted to better understand the intellectual background and the social laboratory-like conditions that led, in Peckham, to the "genesis and development" of the scientific facts of "social self-organization" and "self-responsibility".[17]

"Peckham" as a social generator of knowledge

I have thus tried to penetrate the layers of reception of the Peckham Experiment and obtain a more detailed picture of the centre's founding idea, research practices and everyday reality. All three aspects are amenable to reconstruction with the help of archival materials. A portion of the papers of Scott Williamson and Pearse and a large number of documents produced as the centre went about its business can be viewed at the Wellcome Library for the History of Medicine in London.[18] My examination of these and other supplementary source materials revealed that the Peckham Experiment is by no means "timeless". We can easily trace its founders' motives back to the discourses of social welfare and social medicine of the 1920s. For example, many actors long understood the foundation of the centre as a reform that promised to enhance the fitness of the

British nation. Its directors' hopes of arousing users' initiative differed little from the impetus underlying the moralizing social work already widely practised in the late nineteenth century. And to a certain extent we can account for the enlarged perspective – so surprising at first sight – adopted by physicians Scott Williamson and Pearse, which incorporated aspects of social interaction and integration, if we consider it in light of both the reworking of "reform eugenics" and the theories of evolutionary biology so central to the so-called scientific humanism of the 1930s.

If we pay attention to these contexts we quickly notice that the present-day political debate on the centre, alluded to above, fails to consider how much the Peckham researchers tended to naturalize human behaviour – not least gender relations. This makes their ideas a poor source of concrete social policy proposals for the present. Unfortunately, as yet the scholarly research has shown little interest in the genesis and evolution, over the course of the experiment, of the knowledge for which "Peckham" is now known (or in how, exactly, this knowledge emerged and changed). This research relies overwhelmingly on the published statements of Pearse and Scott Williamson, which often entail retrospective idealization. Accordingly, scholars have created the impression that the centre's "governmental" effects, which they tend to take for granted rather than demonstrate, were intended from the outset. This in turn makes the Peckham scientists seem like strategists of a new type of power relations. Users' pertinacity, room for manoeuvre and contribution, meanwhile, remain obscure.

In what follows, rather than seeking to bring out the timelessness of the Peckham Experiment, I try to shed light on the complications that emerged whenever experts in the social and human sciences sought to put their expertise into practice. Here we need to keep in mind that these complications quite often engendered adaptive pressures that then formed the basis for new insights.[19] The approach adopted by the present book, then, may be understood as a species of historical anthropology centred on the history of knowledge. From a micro-historical vantage point it reconstructs a situation of social interaction that played a part in the genesis (and dissemination) of new knowledge about human beings. I will contextualize this situation as precisely as possible, that is, elucidate the factors leading to the encounter between "biologists" and "guinea pigs", in the spring of 1935, in the premises of a concrete-and-glass building in South London. But the focus then shifts chiefly to the unexpected social occurrences thrown up by this encounter, partly as a consequence of the theories that the scholars brought with them to the centre. Finally, I scrutinize the pressure to generate meaning that was triggered by the behaviour of the centre members. At issue here is the knowledge to which this pressure gave rise – and the covert effect exercised by this knowledge ever since within the broadest range of intellectual and applied contexts.

My epistemological interest, then, is to some extent that of the social historian: its object is an encounter between human beings who belonged to differing social formations, namely activists and scholars of the educated middle classes on the one hand, and members of a milieu centred on crafts-men and skilled labourers on the other. But I have opted not to write the history of the centre primarily as a case study of such an encounter or to foreground its significance to the citizens involved. While a bourgeois habitus serves more than once in what follows as an explanation for Pearse's and Scott Williamson's ways of seeing and behaving, the Peckham Experiment does not provide a representative example of speech acts and strategies typical of a British elite as it sought to affirm itself. In fact it serves better as an example of a certain decline in the "social meaning" (Pierre Bourdieu) of the category of "class"; a shift that, in the case of Peckham, engendered the above-mentioned naturalization of human interaction. However, this by no means made the centre the hierarchy-free space it is often described as.

Structure of the book

Before I can elucidate this naturalization of social relations in more detail, it is vital to place the scholars' engagement and research interest against the back-ground of the heterogeneous health policy landscape of the United Kingdom prior to the establishment of the NHS. Health policy was situated between an ideology of self-help and calls for universal access to medical services, calls that attracted a fair degree of support, particularly in London. Chapter 2 explores these issues by describing the backdrop to the establishment of the first, smaller centre on the Queen's Road and reconstructing the social work performed there between 1926 and 1929. It also provides *biographical information* on Pearse and Scott Williamson and a reading of their programmatic essay, *The Case for Action*, published in 1931.

Chapter 3 then briefly describes the *architecture* of the new centre on St Mary's Road, opened in 1935, while also depicting the first *routines* emerging within it. Having described the initial situation, Chapter 4 moves forward in time and is entirely devoted to the *most-read publication* on the centre, the monograph *The Peckham Experiment*, published in 1943. This is intended to illuminate just how strongly the researchers' interests had shifted in just a short period of time: the "biology" of human interactions itself had now become the object of their attention, reflecting broader intellectual debates of the day on evolution and society.

Chapter 5, however, shows that it is not just the history of ideas that explains the reinterpretation of the centre by Pearse and Scott Williamson. This chapter remains in the second half of the 1930s in order, with the help of memoirs, letters and reports generated by the centre, to look more closely at the research *practices* occurring within it. These too changed significantly as a consequence of a reality shock triggered by Peckham residents' unexpected behaviours.

A brief *summary* (Chapter 6) is then followed by two thematic chapters clearly set apart from the book's chronology. Chapter 7 concerns itself with the *photographs* (and one film) made in and of the centre. Chapter 8 turns to the *users* and their perspective on the experiment. As luck would have it there is plenty of source material to draw on here. This chapter, however, will also show that users' statements do not represent a straightforward corrective to the directors' perspective. In fact, conflicts arose because certain members sought to enforce the researchers' ideas as norms within the centre.

The first part of the book, then, considers the actions and interpretations of as many individuals directly involved in the experiment as possible. But it also tries to show why the legend of Peckham, described at the beginning of the book, took hold. The second part of the book delves more deeply into the reception history of this legend since the 1940s. To this end I draw on a number of sources: press reports, accounts by visitors, and documents produced by various authorities and experts who assessed the centre. Here my account shifts from the local historical micro-level to a discourse-historical macro-level. First, Chapter 9 resumes the previous chronology and explores the period following the centre's closure at the start of the Second World War until it was reopened in 1946. During this period Pearse and Scott Williamson rose to the status of popular *experts* within the debate on the future organization of the British health care system.

Chapter 10 then sheds light on the years from 1946 onwards, exploring the key events that occurred prior to the centre's definitive *closure* in 1950. It clarifies why, just a short while later, the centre seemed quite incapable of surviving into the future. Chapter 11 briefly examines participants' activities subsequent to the experiment, particularly a number of *attempts to re-establish it*, while Chapter 12 provides a *preliminary conclusion*.

Chapter 13, which is the one most concerned with its aftermath, presents *rediscoveries and reinterpretations* of the project since the 1950s in various fields of knowledge. At issue here is the resonance of "Peckham" in anarchists' political theories, in post-war pedagogical thought and, not least, in debates among the architectural and urban planning avant-garde. Above all, though, this concluding chapter shows that in the mid 1940s, in other words when the ideas of Scott Williamson and Pearse attained their maximum spread, social psychologists' interactional experiments generated very similar insights to those of the London-based researchers. Some were in fact influenced by the Peckham Experiment. This provides an opportunity to contemplate to what extent the practice and imagery of the social experiment have played a part in a process we might call the anthropologization of the exploratory life: I argue that the process of experimenting with self-organization and personal responsibility, which I seek to elucidate through the example of the Pioneer Health Centre, gave rise to a vision of the human being as one that constantly explores its own potential, with no certainty about the outcome.

Notes

1 George Scott Williamson and Innes H. Pearse, *The Case for Action. A Survey of Everyday Life under Modern Industrial Conditions, with Special Reference to the Question of Health* (London: Faber & Faber, 1931); George Scott Williamson and

Innes H. Pearse, *Biologists in Search of Material. An Interim Report on the Work of the Pioneer Health Centre, Peckham* (London: Faber & Faber, 1938); Innes H. Pearse and Lucy H. Crocker, *The Peckham Experiment. A Study of the* Living *Structure of Society* (London: Allen & Unwin, 1943); George Scott Williamson, *Physician, Heal Thyself: A Study of Needs and Means* (London: Faber & Faber, 1945); Innes H. Pearse and George Scott Williamson, *Science, Synthesis and Sanity. An Enquiry into the Nature of Living* (London: Collins, 1965); Innes H. Pearse: *The Quality of Life: The Peckham Approach to Human Ethology* (Edinburgh Scottish Academic Press, 1979).

2 "BBC Four. Timeshift", www.bbc.co.uk/programmes/b01mytsg (accessed December 17, 2017). The only one to challenge this narrative is Philip Conford, "'Smashed by the National Health?' A Closer Look at the Demise of the Pioneer Health Centre, Peckham", *Medical History* 60, no. 2 (2016): 250–269.

3 Colin Ward, "Peckham Recollected", *Anarchy* 6 (1966): 52.

4 Axel Scott-Samuel, *Total Participation, Total Health: Reinventing the Peckham Health Centre for the 1990's* (Edinburgh: Scottish Academic Press, 1990).

5 Jonathan Freedland, "Ministers Seeking Inspiration Should Talk to Pam about Prewar Peckham", *The Guardian* (October 31, 2007).

6 For a critical take on Freedland, see: Mike Cushman, "The Peckham Experiment and Other Lost Opportunities", *The Guardian* (November 11, 2007).

7 www.guardian.co.uk/commentisfree/2007/oct/31/comment.politics1 (accessed December 17, 2017).

8 This also goes for the website of the Pioneer Health Foundation, successor to the original organizers of the centre, which continues to promote the Peckham principle: "The Pioneer Health Foundation", www.thephf.org (accessed December 17, 2017). About ten years ago, a special issue of *Social Medicine* (2009, 4, no. 3) underlined the ongoing significance of the PHC. Most recently Emily Charkin has brought the PHC into play as a template for the controversial private "free schools" approved by the Conservative government in 2010: Emily Charkin, "For a Real Free School Look to Postwar Peckham", *The Guardian* (August 30, 2011).

9 For an account that is still worth reading, see: Nikolas Rose, *Powers of Freedom: Reframing Political Thought* (Cambridge: Cambridge University Press, 1999).

10 For an English-language overview of the recent German sociological critique of capitalism, see: Klaus Dörre, Stephan Lessenich and Hartmut Rosa, *Sociology, Capitalism, Critique* (London/New York: Verso, 2015).

11 Ulrich Bröckling, Susanne Krasmann and Thomas Lemke, "From Foucault's Lectures at the Collège de France to Studies of Governmentality. An Introduction", in *Governmentality. Current Issues and Future Challenges*, ed. Ulrich Bröckling, Susanne Krasmann and Thomas Lemke (London: Routledge, 2011), 1–33.

12 Roy Kozlovsky, *The Architectures of Childhood. Children, Modern Architecture and Reconstruction in Postwar England* (London: Routledge, 2013): chapter 1. A similar thesis is presented by: Pyrs Gruffudd, "'Science and the Stuff of Life'. Modernist Health Centres in 1930s London", *Journal of Historical Geography* 27 (2001): 395–416. Of recent research on the PHC, see also: Abigail Beach, "Potential For Participation: Health Centres and the Idea of Citizenship c. 1920–1940", in *Regenerating England. Science, Medicine and Culture in Interwar-Britain*, ed. Christopher Lawrence and Anna K. Mayer (Amsterdam: Rodopi, 2000), 203–230; Emily Charkin, *"He Swings Where There is Space": Education, Freedom and Community at the Peckham Health Centre 1945–1950* (MA thesis, Institute of Education, University of London, 2010); Conford, "'Smashed by the National Health?'", Elizabeth Darling, *Reforming Britain: Narratives of Modernity before Reconstruction* (London: Routledge, 2006).

13 The context of its emergence is described by: Essylt Jones, "Nothing Too Good for the People. Local Labour and London's Interwar Health Centre Movement", *Social History of Medicine* 25 (2012): 84–102.

14 Darling, *Reforming Britain*, 79.
15 This applies in particular to James C. Scott, *Seeing Like a State: How Certain Schemes to Improve the Human Condition Have Failed* (New Haven, Conn./ London: Yale University Press, 1998); and Ulrich Herbert, "Europe in High Modernity. Reflections on a Theory of the 20th Century", *Journal of Modern European History* 5, no. 1 (2007): 5–21.
16 See David Kuchenbuch, *Geordnete Gemeinschaft. Architekten als Sozialingenieure – Deutschland und Schweden im 20. Jahrhundert* (Bielefeld: Transcript, 2010); and Thomas Etzemüller, *Alva and Gunnar Myrdal: Social Engineering in the Modern World* (Lanham: Lexington Books, 2014).
17 Ludwik Fleck, *Genesis and Development of a Scientific Fact* (Chicago: University of Chicago Press, 1981).
18 On its holdings and history of accession, see: Lesley A. Hall, "The Archives of the Pioneer Health Centre, Peckham, in the Wellcome Library", *Social History of Medicine* 14 (2001): 525–538.
19 Lutz Raphael, "Embedding the Human and Social Sciences in Western Societies, 1880–1980", in *Engineering Society. The Role of the Human and Social Sciences in Modern Societies 1880–1980*, ed. by Kerstin Brückweh et al. (Basingstoke: Palgrave Macmillan, 2012), 41–58.

2 From C3 to A1

Reforming the working-class family (1925–1931)

We have to proceed chronologically if we want to know how the Pioneer Health Centre gave rise to the Peckham Experiment. What we quickly discover is that the initiative to establish the centre did not come from the individuals with which it is linked today, George Scott Williamson and Innes Hope Pearse. The actual founders of the centre were classical philanthropists. This is evident in the memoirs, recorded in 1998, of Iris Montagu, wife of the judge and later secret service agent Ewen Montagu, son of an influential banking family. According to her, Dorrit Schlesinger, heir to the van den Bergh soap and margarine producers (whose business was later absorbed into Unilever), had begun to concern herself with the topic of family planning in the early 1920s. Her interest revolved around a classical issue in "positive" eugenics: how one might help the lower classes to consider carefully whether or not to have children, which also meant giving them access to contraception. Together with her husband, the banker Gerald Schlesinger, the Montagus and other interested parties, she set up a committee called South West Welfare that was meant to explore relevant educational methods in practice, initially in West London. In order to shed light on the medical dimension as well, the group made contact with paediatrician Alice Model, who then recommended Pearse. She in turn proposed getting Scott Williamson on board; she was his assistant at the time. The group began to amass funds; the Schlesingers as well as John Benjamin Sainsbury, son of the founder of the supermarket chain of the same name, were particularly generous donors, as was Jack (John George Stuart) Donaldson, later minister for the arts and Baron Donaldson of Kingsbridge, and his future wife Frances Lonsdale, who joined the group shortly afterwards.[1]

The Peckham Experiment, then, resembles the many civilizing missions launched by bourgeois reformers in the "darker" corners of the metropolis. We are dealing here with prosperous philanthropists motivated by concern for the national resource of "population". City dwellers in particular no longer seemed to reproduce on a "natural" scale; in general the city was home to the cumulative negative effects of modernization. Urbanization appeared to bring social segregation in its wake, particularly the migration of the well-to-do to the suburbs. The group, therefore, saw itself in part as the modern equivalent of the traditional country doctor. On this view, the latter was able to guarantee not just personal care and corresponding early diagnosis but also ensured the social cohesion of the British people. The founders' main focus, however, was on the children of the urban lower classes, who represented the "wealth of nations", as a 1925 memorandum put it. Governments across the world, they believed, were only just beginning to appreciate "that there is no room for the useless member of society and that the unhealthy citizen is merely a burden on the family and the state; they realise, further, that the healthy child generally develops into a healthy man or woman and that a healthy citizen is always an asset to the country".[2]

Contemporary welfarist strategies, they contended, while humanitarian, were not geared towards the future. This was because they ignored the fact that healthy and useful citizens could only develop in intact families. Among the working classes especially, they pointed out, pregnancies were often unplanned, with very little attention being paid to the health risks involved. So it was all the more crucial to involve individuals from this section of the population – both intellectually and emotionally – in efforts to enhance their living conditions. It was particularly important to forge contact with young couples who were still amenable to influence: "We must [...] develop their inherent sense of responsibility; we must implant in their minds how essential it is for them to be in a fit state themselves before they contemplate the creation of life."[3] A leisure centre would be the ideal way of doing so. It would, the founders were convinced, make it possible to pursue social work through regular contact with the whole family. One could lure them in by exploiting their "inherent desire for some constructive hobby". The centre could, for example, provide tools (for the men) and cooking utensils (for the women):

> The Medical staff will take advantage of their intimacy with the parents to impress upon them the value of such Public Health matters as Vaccination, Dental Prophylaxis, the Shick test for Diphtheria and other modern advancements of proved value in preventive medicine.

These remarks culminate in the slogan:

> Peaceful homes
> Happy parenthood
> Healthy babies
> Useful citizenship.[4]

When this text was composed the founders had already contacted the LCC and obtained approval from the Ministry of Health to initiate the project.[5] And they had found a site for it, a two-storey Victorian terraced house with a garden at 142 Queen's Road, the main street in Peckham, just a stone's throw from Queen's Road Peckham, one of the smaller stops on the railway line running through the district of Southwark in South London. Gerald Schlesinger paid the lion's share of the purchase price of £1,600 for the site and the building, which seemed perfectly located for the project. It was occupying a central position within an area that was not plagued by poverty – with a population that consisted mostly of craftsmen and skilled labourers and their families – and, importantly, not entirely lacking in social institutions, making it possible to test out the attraction of a centre based on voluntary membership. A number of repairs were made, medical equipment was acquired, and the association gave itself an administrative structure. Important decisions were made by the General Committee, which met once a year, while the Executive Committee dealt with everyday matters and a four-person Working Staff took care of the day-to-day running of the centre.[6]

On Queen's Road

The new institution opened in 1926. There are no user memoirs or other ego-documents from this period so we have to reconstruct everyday life at the centre with the help of its annual reports, which tend to be rather rose-tinted, being intended for the centre's supporters, the so-called subscribers. It was in this publication, in late 1926, that Dorrit Schlesinger described the centre's first few months. This she did – establishing a technique that was to be used into the 1970s – by describing the premises from the perspective of a visitor, thus allowing chance encounters to speak for themselves.

The door opens and the reader is met by the resident secretary, Mrs Reid, who immediately asks whether he would like to become a member – only those living in the immediate vicinity of Queen's Road, she explains, can use the centre. Reid loses no time in presenting the premises underlying the project: "[E]ducational work, we consider, cannot be a matter of general propaganda, it must be a matter of personal and individual contact." The reader enters the former living room, now the club room (Figure 2.1), taking in the brand-new sewing machines. A cards night will be held later that day, providing an opportunity to mention another special feature of the centre: everything costs money. There are no patients, only members, as: "One of our chief aims is to teach our members to shoulder the responsibility of their own health." Making his way down the stairs to the consulting room, the reader encounters Pearse, resident medical officer, who is in the process of weighing a baby. There is time for a glance at the garden, where Mrs Holland is keeping an eye on several young children and you notice a shed with a workbench for the men.[7]

Pearse's medical report strikes a more impersonal tone than Schlesinger's walkabout. At the centre, it states, information on infant care and contraception is provided in a relaxed, informal manner. At the same time the institution seeks to combat the disintegration of the family, allowing parents time for one another as someone else supervises their children and keeps them busy. Pearse also mentions a health overhaul, a routine medical investigation

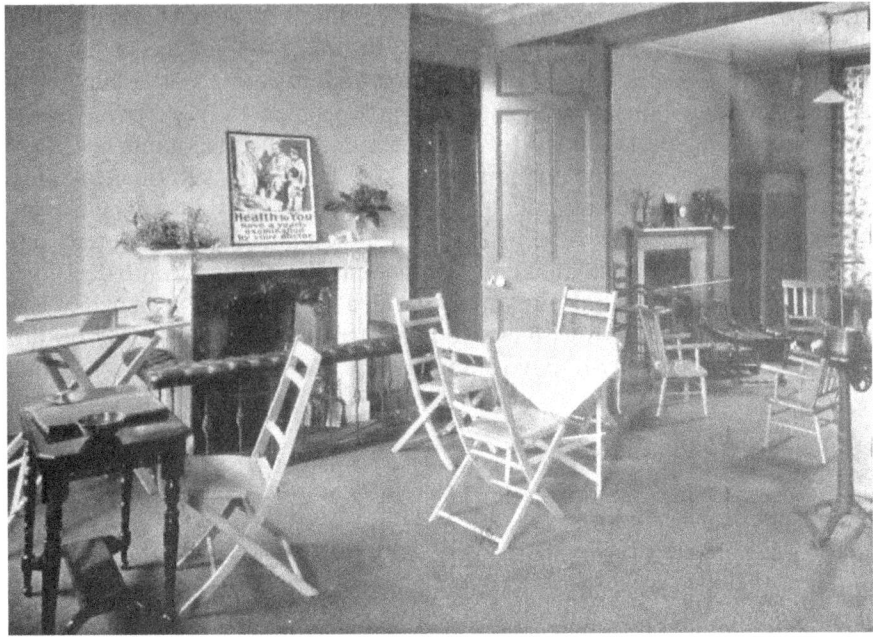

Figure 2.1 Club room of the centre on Queen's Road, from the annual report of 1926 (WL, SA/PHC/A.2/1)

that helps assess the state of users' health. In the first year alone, it is claimed, this has brought to light more than 100 previously undiagnosed illnesses.[8]

The next annual report in 1927 was already able to announce that the centre's membership was growing at a pleasingly fast rate. It had, the report continued, therefore become necessary to erect an annex in the garden in order to create space for a viable nursery (for the afternoons), and for events such as boxing matches and dance nights. The centre's popularity, according to the report, had enabled it to provide a great deal of advice of many different kinds, which was already having an effect. The second examination of all members after one year had revealed significant improvements in the state of their health. They were paying more attention to hygiene; many adults had been persuaded to visit the dentist; and the children were being breastfed more often, partly because Scott Williamson was promoting the practice in his "chats" with fathers.[9] The same year, he hailed the centre as a comprehensive success: almost 80 families were now frequenting it. Scott Williamson reported that plans were afoot to sell beer – an unusual measure given the moralism of many welfare institutions at the time. This step was intended to bind the men more tightly to the centre; though many of them, he wrote, went there to play cards after work, later they moved on to the pub.[10] Scott Williamson also complained that the centre was bursting at the seams. Many families were abandoning it because of the overcrowding. The outline of a comprehensive solution to social problems was beginning to emerge, but the building was impeding attempts to gain a more precise understanding of it. The project risked becoming a victim of its own success.[11]

But Scott Williamson was rather vague about what, precisely, the centre promised to achieve. The sources of the time provide us with the very little evidence of the phenomenon so central to the centre's later reception: social self-organization. The statements made during this phase generally come across as surprisingly paternalistic. There is much talk of education, with the residents of Peckham appearing as passive recipients of guidance and character-building:

> To take children of working class parents who are ignorant or careless and to attend to the health and early upbringing of those children is doing fine work for humanity and for civilization. But to take those *parents* also and shew them how to *give* that very attention, and *why* they should do so, is far finer work, and far more *efficacious* in the long run. The idea of Welfare Work should not merely be to *relieve* the working classes of their responsibilities towards their children, but rather to teach them those responsibilities for themselves.[12]

Pioneers?

The PHC, then, by no means started out as a large-scale research project. Initially, even medical screening played a merely minor role. It served to evaluate the effects of the social work carried out within the centre, and was also intended to attract families who could avail themselves of a low-cost examination (but not treatment). In the 1920s the health centre was run on a voluntary basis and had a specific agenda centred on population policy – and as such it was not especially original.

At this point we could spend a lot of time delving into the tremendous anxiety over the general population's health, productivity and reproductive capacity felt in many industrial societies in the first decades of the twentieth century. The state took it upon itself to improve the so-called public health in order to bolster the nation's – and, often, the race's – military clout and economic competitiveness; this was also intended to keep down the costs of the nascent system of social insurance. Much has been written about key actors' increasingly "medicalized" (Ivan Illich) perspective on the population and approach to individuals, and there have been plenty of accounts of the associated "bio-power" (Michel Foucault). Both comparatively mild educational practices and harsher governmental interventions pursued for medical reasons always sought to enforce social mores or norms of productivity. This applied especially in cases in which, in one way or another, the individual body seemed to risk infecting, in both moral and physiological terms, the societal whole or nation. The national or collective body, it was feared, was at latent risk of degeneration, and the large city was seen as the most dangerous place in this respect.[13] It was no novelty for social medicine and social hygiene to create expectations about how certain social groups ought to behave, with respect, for example, to the expenditure and regeneration of energy in their "human motor", their bodily care, their dwelling practices and their sexual behaviour.[14]

But neither were the founders the first to come up with the more specific idea of creating a local drop-in centre for medical advice. Despite their later claims, they certainly did not coin the term "health centre". The "pioneer" tag belies the fact that in Britain health centres had been discussed – even on the governmental level – for years before the opening of the centre on Queen's Road. Most prominently, the so-called Dawson Report, published in 1920, had proposed a national network of health centres. These were conceived as institutions that would house a number of general practitioners and provide primary care. Minor operations could be carried out, and they would also offer so-called physical culture services such as sports equipment.[15] Subsequently, the concept of the health centre in fact became the lowest common denominator of quite different political groupings. For example, in a series of programmatic texts of the 1920s and early 1930s the Socialist Medical Association (SMA) embraced the concept in association with demands for a nationwide "socialized" health care system.[16]

With its focus on ensuring that the next generation was of the "best" quality, the Queen's Road centre has to be seen in the light of widespread concerns about the health of the "children of the poor". This theme was central to social policy debates in the UK, with scholarly publications and political lobbying groups beginning to focus on the topic at the turn of the century.[17] It became more urgent with the mustering of recruits for the Second Boer War (1899–1902). This brought to light a large number of young men categorized as "C3", in other words who seemed unfit to go to war – most of them as a result of deficiency diseases such as rickets, which were in turn traced back to social circumstances. The recruits' wretched physical condition was an effect of poverty, whose appalling scale was publicized around the same time by texts such as Benjamin Seebohm Rowntree's first study of York (1901) and, a little later, the survey *Round About a Pound a Week* (1913).[18] Particularly in London, a culture of statistical studies that first emerged around the turn of the century continued to grow in importance after the First World War, engendering a new awareness of the (poor) living and nutritional standards of a large portion of the urban populace.[19] All this culminated in the demand for measures to improve "national efficiency", if not for the "regeneration" of Britain and the British Empire.[20]

By 1911 an initial, compulsory form of health insurance for low earners had been established through the National Insurance Act. This, however, covered a limited range of benefits, and by the 1930s the government had already made cuts – in comparative European perspective, the British health care system long remained patchy and the individual's health care continued to depend largely on factors such as income, the particular insurance scheme involved, age, gender and place of residence.[21] Nonetheless, in 1919 the debates on reform prompted the establishment of the Ministry of Health under the ever-busy George Newman, who introduced compulsory medical examinations in schools and promoted school sports.[22] A year earlier the passing of the Maternity and Child Welfare Act triggered the establishment of a number of welfare centres, which provided services similar to those of the PHC. The centre's foundation, then, was enmeshed with broad debates on the social causes of disease and the methods of both social medicine and health education. At the time of the founding of the Queen's Road centre a number of pressure groups were already promoting preventative medicine, and in 1927 they banded together to form the Central Council for Health Education,[23] while periodicals such as *New Health* and *Better Health* propagated improved eating habits and sporting activity. Finally, "keep fit" was the slogan of the National Fitness Campaign initiated by the government in the early 1930s, which urged the British people to embrace preventative practices with the help of propaganda films and posters.[24]

Helping with self-help

At most, then, the Pioneer Health Centre was one of many pioneering projects within the heterogeneous health policy landscape of its founding era. In fact, the institution that Scott Williamson began to present as a crucial innovation from the late 1920s onwards seems anything but "modern" when we consider how little its founders initially did to mask their bourgeois sense of superiority. Their assumption that it was necessary to educate city dwellers to take responsibility for themselves inevitably recalls the settlement houses that shot up in many countries in the late nineteenth century. In the UK this occurred chiefly in the East End of London, but also in the vicinity of Peckham. The settlement movement was propelled by the conviction that closer everyday contact between the "lower" and "educated classes" would help achieve social peace and bolster national cohesion. Viewed from another angle, the settlement houses may thus be regarded as sites of bourgeois identity formation, where an elite sought to affirm the universality of its educational ideals and ethic of achievement by imparting them to others.[25] Although it did not focus on the poorest social stratum per se, it cannot be ignored that the PHC – in its earliest incarnation – featured remnants of a notion of self-help typical of the Victorian age. For many Victorian reformers, poverty was an expression of individuals' lack of will to overcome their problems and take responsibility for their own lives.[26] The neo-Gladstonians and philanthropists who banded together in the Charity Organisation Society (COS), for instance, thus insisted on the principle of subsidiarity.[27] Social work must take account of the singularity of the afflicted's problems – of an essentially spiritual and moral nature – which were impeding their successful participation in the job market. This was one of the reasons why they advocated an emphatic localism when it came to the practice of helping people.

This practice, moreover, seemed capable of helping stabilize family relationships, partly as a means of averting old-age poverty. The COS rejected the idea of anonymous charity, but was particularly dismissive of government benefits. The latter – unlike the friendly societies, which the COS welcomed – seemed inefficient, but also unethical due to their materialism.

We can trace this attitude into the famous *Majority Report* of the Royal Commission on the Poor Laws and Relief of Distress, published in 1909, which sought to assess the Poor Law legislation. More influential over the long term, however, was the *Minority Report*, compiled under the auspices of Beatrice and Sidney Webb, who were active in the reform socialist Fabian Society. As in many other European countries, in the United Kingdom too the scientization of social policy began to set in around the turn of the century, not least because social policy was reconceptualized as a response to the risk calculations generated by actuarial mathematics.[28] For the Webbs and their fellow campaigners poverty was rooted in socioeconomic relations of dependency.[29] Their perspective – oversimplifying somewhat – had less to do with problematizing the morality of the pauper than with acknowledging the structural character of poverty, which had earlier been given striking visual expression in Charles Booth's poverty maps of London. That said, if we look at the measures recommended in the *Minority Report* we find plenty of room for hybrid solutions. In 1909 the Webbs had nothing against private organizations providing donation-funded welfare benefits, as long as they did not compete with public institutions. Especially when it came to special cases of poverty (as with the mentally ill or orphans), they regarded such initiatives as more organizationally agile. They expressed support for so-called "pioneer experiments" partly in light of the modern sciences' tendency for specialization, which might be impeded by the sluggish state.[30]

So to some extent at least the centre on Queen's Road – unsurprisingly given its initiators' social position – seems to have perpetuated the self-help paradigms of the late nineteenth century in light of medical imperatives. Set against the debates of the day, the goal of familiarizing oneself with individual families' living conditions in order to influence them positively was not particularly progressive. This is evident if we take the local political context into account. After the 1929 Local Government Act, which enabled the LCC to take charge of Poor Law institutions (such as hospitals, which previously accepted patients only after assessing their eligibility), the London Labour Party (LLP) committed itself to an emphatically egalitarian health policy, while criticizing – far more sharply than the Webbs – the class differences and organizational redundancies reproduced (or caused) by the voluntary sector in London.[31]

If anything, what was novel about the centre in Peckham – though quite uncontroversial given the general interest in social medicine – was the idea of evaluating scientifically the effectiveness of an informal approach to providing medical advice. In 1925 this scientific project was still anchored in the hope that generalizable methods would be found to help young working-class families make rational decisions about whether to have children. Little by little, however, the Peckham researchers' interests shifted to the micro-structural conditions that made such responsible decisions possible in the first place. They began to pay attention to the social sphere as such, or to be more precise, to the dynamics of interpersonal relations within an individual's immediate environment.

Biographical aspects

At this point it is useful to survey the biographies of the centre's later directors, who were responsible for this shift.[32] Comprehensive literary remains are available neither for Pearse nor Scott Williamson; the only biographical material we have for them exists in the form of curriculum vitae.[33] George Scott Williamson was born in 1884 (1883 according to some obituaries) as the son of a minister and the oldest of seven children in Ladybank, north of Edinburgh. Scott Williamson, called "Dod" by his friends and "Doc Willy" or simply "Doc" by many users of the centre,[34] began his medical studies in 1904 at the Edinburgh School of Medicine, graduating in 1906 as Bachelor of Medicine and Bachelor of Surgery. After his studies he first worked at the Greenwich Poor Law Asylum,[35] then from 1908 at the research laboratory of the West Riding Lunatic Asylum, a psychiatric institution in Yorkshire. From 1910 to 1919 he carried out research as a pathologist at the University of Bristol. Despite his encounter with poverty, at this point in time he was by no means a liberal reformer: Scott Williamson organized a protest by a number of doctors against the new system of health insurance in Bristol in 1911 – evidently, this was the only emphatically political activity in which he had ever been involved.[36] During the First World War he was stationed in France with the Royal Army Medical Corps. Here, as lieutenant-colonel, he rendered out-standing services organizing a field hospital in Étretat in Normandy – which is interesting in light of his later activity as director of an establishment in which *nothing* was organized. He was "Mentioned in Dispatches" in recognition of his contribution and was captured by German forces in 1917.[37] From 1920 on, overlapping with the period when he began his work in Peckham, he worked as a pathologist at the Royal Free Hospital in the City of London, an old phi-lanthropic establishment that had treated the "deserving poor" free of charge since the mid nineteenth century. Here, mostly with the help of scholarships, he carried out research on pathologies of the thyroid. He also gave his first lectures at institutions such as the Royal College of Surgeons.

Pearse and Scott Williamson married in 1950. He died just three years later without completing his magnum opus, on which he had been working since 1939. He left behind a copious bundle of draft chapters, which Pearse turned into the book *Science, Synthesis and Sanity*, published posthumously in 1969. A few years later, Pearse published her own simplified version of his ideas, entitled *The Quality of Life*. In the appendix to this book we find a number of "flashbacks" from Scott Williamson's life. Here he tells of how, as a child, he had attended to his brother, who was suffering from tuberculosis, without becoming infected. Prior to his studies, he stated, he had witnessed a smallpox epidemic on a quarantine ship, where he had seen a terminally ill woman give birth to a completely healthy baby by Caesarean section. From then on, he claimed, insusceptibility to infection had been the dominant theme of his life.[38] Otherwise it is hard to find out anything about Scott Williamson. He was supposed to become a minister, he liked reading detective novels, had some experience of theosophy, believed in some sort of mystical "cosmos", but was not religious in the conventional sense.[39] Other sources tell us that he was generous with other people's property and had unhealthy habits: apparently he was a chain smoker who rarely left the house.[40]

There is even less information available on Pearse ("Pete"). And yet her career as a long-unmarried, working woman with a university degree is a remarkable one. Innes Hope Pearse was born in 1889, completed her higher education at the London Medical School for Women and Royal Free Hospital and obtained her degree in 1916. She took up a post at the Bristol Royal Hospital for Women and Children, which she later described as a frustrating but crucial experience. Here, she explained, she had learned nothing about the living conditions of sick children and had never set eyes on healthy children in order, as it were, to make comparisons.[41] In 1918 she worked as a doctor at the Great Northern Hospital in London; from 1919 at the London Hospital; in 1920 she taught at St Thomas's Hospital, also in London, and from 1921 to 1935, with a number of interruptions, she then worked as assistant to Scott Williamson at the Free Hospital. Evidently, she had previously had to abandon her desire to become a surgeon due to illness. From 1925 she initially worked in Peckham in parallel to her work in the hospital, and then on a full-time basis from 1935 to 1939 and 1946 to 1950. During the Second World War, together with her colleague Lucy Crocker, she wrote probably the most widely read book on the centre, *The Peckham Experiment*. After Scott Williamson's death her work consisted in efforts to initiate new institutions based on the centre.[42] *The Quality of Life* appeared in 1979, shortly after her death on December 28, 1978.

Finally, we have virtually nothing to go on when it comes to the relationship between Scott Williamson and Pearse. At any rate the pair married after around 30 years of close collaboration. Apparently, however, they never presented themselves to centre members as a couple, which is odd in light of the familial ideology that pervades their publications. Nor did they have any children. Only by reading between the lines do we discover that the two physicians – very unusually for the era – were already living together unmarried in the 1940s (in 1941 in Bishop's Stortford to the north of London, in 1943 in the posh Hyde Park Mansions in West London and later in suburban Bromley), at certain times together with other members of centre staff.[43] What is certain is that Scott Williamson's and Pearse's tasks at the centre were gender-based. In the first few years in particular, Pearse mainly practised paediatrics. Scott Williamson's job description was more vague. Other members of staff seem to have perceived Pearse, who was more reserved than her extrovert partner, as something of the aloof scientist, while "Doc Willy" was the jovial free spirit.[44] Apparently, Scott

Williamson repeatedly urged Pearse to drop her stuffy persona: "He would say 'use your eyes, woman, and see what's going on around you. Don't just go through the routine and put it all down on paper.'"[45] As audio documents reveal, Pearse spoke a pronounced upper-class English.[46]

At this point it is important to mention that in the early 1930s the two physicians' medical work in a narrower sense attracted a degree of controversy. Scott Williamson appears to have been a charismatic, enthusiastic scientist, but one who was not always overly meticulous. This is evident in documents from the Medical Research Council (MRC), the UK's leading state funding body for medical research (founded in 1913), to which he applied in 1929 requesting a scholarship for Pearse. These documents reveal that orthodox histologists were sceptical about Scott Williamson's research on the thyroid.[47] A confidential letter by an MRC expert to its president, Walter Morley Fletcher, even stated:

> [Scott Williamson] seems to lack training in exact scientific investigation. Perhaps it is a natural defect of the critical instinct. [...] Like many enthusiasts, he readjusts his theories to new facts, even in the course of a conversation, with rather dangerous agility.[48]

For a time Scott Williamson received the Mackenzie-Mackinnon research scholarship from the Royal College of Surgeons. In 1932 the latter obtained information about him from the MRC, evidently troubled by rumours about his work: "The [...] Committee wants to be quite sure that he is not being carried away in this or that direction."[49] The same year, the Council opted not to renew Pearse's grant.[50] Was the centre partly a means of obtaining employment? Were the researchers now compelled to go for broke because the funding for their thyroid research threatened to run dry? This question is particularly interesting given that at this point in time one of the MRC's key funding priorities was preventative medicine. This became even more important during the time of the second, larger health centre in Peckham, as reflected in the Social Medicine Research Unit founded in the late 1940s.[51]

Plans for expansion

In any event, the building on Queen's Road was closed and sold in 1929. A plot of land for a new building, not far from the old centre, had been secured the year before (Figure 2.2). At the same time the group of people associated with it began to ascribe broad social significance to the observations made at the Queen's Road institution. For example, in a speech to the London League of Nations Union, Dorrit Schlesinger underlined that the centre had shown that peace, health and happiness could not be achieved through "propaganda" but only "by personal individual education".[52] Scott Williamson too began to relate the project's findings to society as a whole, as evident in the title of a 1931 memorandum entitled "Paper on Scientific Enquiry into Social

Disintegration".[53] Another manuscript includes a further, momentous generalization. Here Scott Williamson asserts that the centre's users had not only willingly paid the membership fee but in fact thought it too low. The centre's role as a provider of services rather than charity, he believed, had thus been an important source of its popularity. This in turn proved that in the main people would accept advice if they could regard it not as a mere gift but as something they had paid for: "The parents desired the responsibility of paying for value received."[54] Two years later, in a scholarship application, Scott Williamson wrote: "The Pioneer Health Centre has found a means of inducing the man in the street to feel and to take personal and financial responsibility for the promotion of his health and that of his family."[55] He also suggested here that the centre in Peckham had been successful as a pilot project in economic terms. It had, he contended, demonstrated that the membership fee – which working- and lower middle-class people were willing and able to pay in exchange for medical advice and health-promoting activities – was sufficient to sustain centres such as the PHC. A comprehensive practice of preventative medicine seemed possible even in the absence of expensive state-run programmes.

There are, however, a number of indications that the centre on Queen's Road could by no means cover its running costs from membership fees.[56] One of the main motives for planning a larger centre was clearly the hope that more members would help reduce running costs per head. In 1929 Scott Williamson had calculated that a few research scholarships and a mortgage on the building would be enough to cover the new centre's running costs, indeed to amortize the initial investment[57] – in part because over time the membership fee could be doubled. The idea here was that having once come into contact with the centre, the people of Peckham would no longer spend their money on other (less worthy) leisure activities.[58]

But it was clear that substantial start-up capital would be required. In February 1931, therefore, the charitable venture known as the Pioneer Health Centre Limited was established.[59] It soon began to organize charity balls (in the gardens of Kensington Palace, for example) and commissioned elaborate publicity materials. These directed their pithy slogans at potential donors – virtually every brochure from this period came with a payment slip.[60] Efforts were made in parallel to obtain cheap credit from businesses, with John Sainsbury in particular arguing unashamedly that the money would be going to a project of great utility from a business perspective. The centre, he wrote, would show "that essential social services can be founded on a commercial basis and need not be a drain on Charity, Industry or the Taxpayer".[61]

It is striking that the planned centre's objectives gradually changed in appeals for donations during this period. Initially there was much talk of birth control, applied eugenics and the "C3" population that the centre would help cure. By 1934, however, the appeal, in bold type, for "Healthier Babies!" had vanished from the back cover of the annual reports. Instead a

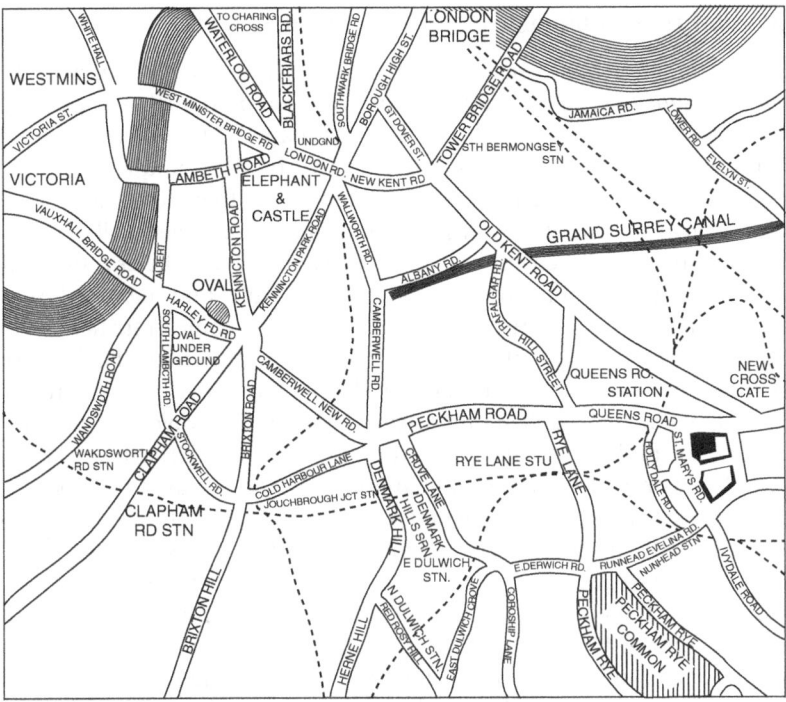

Figure 2.2 Site of the planned new centre in South London featuring local transport options, redrawn from a brochure (c. 1933) (C3 ... or A1?, undated, WL, SA/PHC/B.3/22/3)

brochure announced the new centre grandiloquently as "A new Plan of National Health-Building" that was of vital importance to all taxpayers.[62] Contemporary political references also cropped up. One leaflet alluded to the world economic crisis but warned that it was not the only issue worthy of attention given that the "social life of the nation" was in a state of disarray. We can also discern an anti-communist tone in the same text – the centre guaranteed welfare without bureaucracy and Bolshevism.[63] But the most important change in the way those involved presented their work to the world concerned the history of the closed building on Queen's Road. They now claimed that, right from the start, they had carried out a preliminary experiment, a first step in a larger full experiment.[64] Yet there had been no talk at all of experiments in the 1920s. Back then a flyer had referred to the centre as part of a "Pioneer Movement".[65] At the start of the following decade, for Scott Williamson and Pearse, a movement for the reform of social policy had become a scientific research project, as their first book also lays bare.

Responsibility as a biological function: the first book

The Case for Action. A Survey of Everyday Life under Modern Industrial Conditions, with Special Reference to the Question of Health was published in 1931 by the recently established Faber & Faber. Here Pearse and Scott Williamson developed a multifaceted presentational technique to which they adhered for the rest of their lives: they elaborated their ideas in books of a popular cast that were often downright sentimental and generally included at best rudimentary references to other research. Nonetheless they always ensured that these publications looked respectable and included scientific -elements such as bar charts and tables displaying some statistical material. The titles of these books always repay closer examination. Their 1931 text fused the empirical study ("survey") and interventionist reform programme ("action"), while the subheading suggested that the topic of "health" was merely one example of the study of everyday life in modern industrial society. The two forewords also hamper any attempt to clearly classify the book. First comes a short text by Lord Moynihan. As president of the Royal College of Surgeons he put his full weight behind the study as a *physician*, while also locating it unambiguously within the context of preventative medicine. The second foreword, meanwhile, was by Alexander Dunlop Lindsay, rector of the progressive Balliol College, Oxford, and influential philosopher. For him the book presented a highly promising "social experiment" that upheld the precept that must inspire all sensible social reforms: "the principle of social self-maintenance."[66]

The main text presents familiar ideas in social medicine. The general population's "devitalised" C3 condition, particularly that of recruits, is a national problem, a "waste of human energies". Too few people are fit, and even the best health propaganda can do nothing to change this. But "personal hygiene" cannot be optimized through the anonymous redistribution of resources, which in any case often results in dependency and "spiritual poverty", just like philanthropy. So the question that arises is: "Could the individual be induced to take part in prevention if the opportunity was available?" The centre on Queen's Road, we are told, has not only shown that this is possible. It has also demonstrated that the most effective way of doing so is to encourage people in close relationships to spur each other on, for example by using "'rumour' or 'gossip'" to spread knowledge of hygiene. Pearse and Scott Williamson went so far as to use a word that rarely has positive connotations in medical texts: "By means of infection with ideas and feeling, it was possible to disseminate knowledge and at the same time evoke a desire to act upon it." In order to facilitate this infection, moreover, attempts had been made to dismantle institutional barriers. The expert had presented him- or herself as a "knowledgeable friend" rather than a profes-sional source of authority.[67]

The directors of the centre had then assessed the impact of this approach through annual follow-up examinations.[68] Here, beyond the medical facts, they had learned a great deal about the residents of Peckham.[69] For example, they had noted that as a rule the worker is not "careless and lazy", not the "apathetic individual we are generally led to believe". If you address yourself to the worker in the right way, he is quite willing to accept help in order to achieve "social adjustment". He also has an intuitive sense of physical dysfunctions. But because mere instruction is not enough to prompt him to visit the doctor more regularly, it is all the more important to maintain constant contact with him. This led Pearse and Scott Williamson to make a statement that was anything but self-evident in 1931: "Advice may be given, but it need not be taken."[70] Yet there is no doubt whatsoever which readers the book was addressing, if for strategical reasons: those concerned with the working classes' willingness to behave productively and their capacity to do so.

However, from a rather pragmatic observation – individuals' preventative behaviour can be more effectively enhanced if you include their relatives – *The Case for Action* derives truly fundamental ideas about human capabilities. Pearse and Scott Williamson contend that: "The individual and his environment are inseparable. They are moreover in function reciprocally stimulant." In fact, the greater part of the book portrays different stages of the human life: the pairing process, pregnancy, the growth of children and so on – always anchored in the notion that there is a unique *biological* potential inherent in every human being. This potential is realized according to its own logic, but only in a social environment rich in stimulation. Here Pearse and Scott Williamson emphasize their rejection of the segregation of children according to age group, as typical of the school system. This, they assert, clashes with the specific routes and rhythms that unleash the individual's potential. A far better approach is to ensure that they enjoy a specific "home" – in which new knowledge is filtered through the social "womb" to which the developing human being is accustomed. What they have in mind here is the social community in which the parents' lives are embedded. However, according to the authors this organic integration has regressed in the industrialized societies, not least because urban life and mechanization have stifled women's urge for nest-building.[71] This has endangered the family, the smallest possible environment and the real human organism.[72] Scott Williamson and Pearse, then, naturalize gender difference and social community, embedding both in a kind of developmental theory. An "urge to responsability [sic]" is hereditary in the human being. But rather than being determined, the strength of this drive is shaped by environmental conditions – and can be increased by them. Here we can discern a semantic operation that was to have absurd results in later writings by Scott Williamson. Latin-based composite terms are reinterpreted by foregrounding the meaning of their separate components: *responsibility* becomes "respons-ability" – a biological function the authors compare with the way the semipermeable cell membrane interacts with its environment. Pearse and Scott Williamson regard human social adaptability as an essential biological feature, though one it is crucial to help along if the goal is to stimulate the "growth" of human society as a whole. It is remarkable how they derive – from observations concerning working-class families' capacity for learning – a thesis that could scarcely be more comprehensive: "Responsability [sic] is a biological attribute of consciousness; it is the very essence of health."[73] Their interpretation of the concept of responsibility is radically naturalistic. It no longer has any moral component at all.

It seems as though Scott Williamson and Pearse were reluctant to fully elaborate on their self-confident assertion. Their book goes on to dedicate itself to concrete issues such as the raising of children, soon revealing the normativity of the potential the experts intended to realize. At least some of the "biological" objectives were clear. Scott Williamson and Pearse left no room for doubt that they knew exactly how the energies of growing children and adolescents ought to be channelled, in order, for example, to prevent poor "mentality, manners, and uncouth bearing".[74] It is here that ideological remnants of the settlement movement shine through most clearly, for example when the authors claim that youths should ideally be exposed to a high degree of social mixing, something they lack in the class-segregated, monocultural urban world. Where there is a dearth of stimulation from the environment they will seek it out in artificial ways, for example at the cinema. This gets them overexcited and thus entails the risk that developmental stages will be skipped. The self-image emanating from these passages is typical of many social reformers and social workers in the early twentieth century. They themselves are still the best source of stimulation: "[C]ontinuous individual contact with a better example [...] is the only sure and natural method of which we are aware of stirring the feeling, which alone is capable of giving the necessary urge to action." Overall, according to Pearse and Scott Williamson, they have learned two things from the pilot project. First, close contact between the doctor and the entire family is the best way of sensitizing people to the significance of early diagnosis. Second, of key importance is an insight into the finances of the households of the lower classes: "[T]he artisan is prepared to spend his money in taking responsibility for the maintenance of his own health and that of his family."[75] But the authors are not content with these essentially social policy-related observations. They go on to reinterpret them as facts of life that must be investigated in more detail. Nature itself had begun to oust the Victorian striving for independence and respectability. Personal responsibility had become biological:

> [W]e have seen that responsibility and health are synonymous. [...] Health demands that a man shoulder his own burden. It is better that he receive his whole wage and himself take the responsibility for his own welfare than that he be given what is presumed to be good for him and robbed of responsibility.[76]

Internal supremacy

In their book Scott Williamson and Pearse presented a research programme centred on the optimization of human beings' natural adaptability and capacity for action – though these abilities seemed virtually coterminous with "health". They concluded that a new centre was essential, a place full of knowledge that would provide members with plenty of ways of becoming active. In fact, in 1931 the authors were already planning much of what distinguished the later centre on St Mary's Road. At the end of their book they take us on a tour through an imaginary building featuring a swimming pool and sports equipment, a library, a cafeteria – an edifice that would make it easy for its users to move around freely while also allowing the experts to observe their development in detail. The future "organizers" would become "operators in the gallery of the theatre, directing the spot-light first on one actor, then on the next, as each takes up the responsible action upon the stage of life".[77] This vivid passage is followed by sober reflections on the optimal size of such an ensemble. It must generate sufficient funds from membership fees to cover its running costs. The number of members, meanwhile, must be large enough to deliver statistically significant results. On the other hand, the centre must not become so large and anonymous as to impede personal contact between those in attendance. Overall, this would facilitate a better understanding of the functions of life, and thus help advance the "progressive differentiation" of the species as a whole – by unleashing the human being's *internal* forces:

> Up till the present time the last or "western" civilization has been swayed by ambitions of external dominion. The new epoch that is approaching calls for internal supremacy – *homo* triumphant not over the external world alone but also over his own dual self.[78]

As progressive as this seems, when it comes to the myth of Peckham it is crucial to note that the recreational activities in the planned centre were by no means to be self-administered. On the contrary, the passages describing these activities in *The Case for Action* are defined by the language of organization, discipline, control and education. The nursery, for example, must be the site of "organized games and songs" – activities intended to achieve a "disciplined action of body and mind". The physicians even worked on the assumption that they would test the children's intelligence and convince their parents of the best educational path for their offspring. The reading room too – as a pedagogical site – was of far greater importance than in the centre that was eventually established. It was supposed to feature tutors who would arouse a "legitimate demand for lectures, demonstrations, debates, poetry and dramatic readings, plays, music".[79] Above all, though, there was nothing informal about the members' clubs. In fact they were to be put together following an aptitude test:

Into these intramural clubs each individual, subject to his needs and inclinations, will be drafted by medical prescription at the time of, or subsequent to his medical overhaul. Within each club, graded and balanced teams will measure their skill and progress with one another.[80]

In 1931, then, Scott Williamson and Pearse were still assuming that they could and must optimize users' potential by assessing their performance, by selecting and assorting individuals. They were seriously concerned that they might fritter away their leisure time at the centre: "Thus the intramural clubs [...] will be at the same time a source of disciplined development and not merely a way of whiling away time."[81]

The Case for Action is an idiosyncratic text. It combines ideas that, from a modern-day perspective, do not belong together. It urges its readers to become active, to promote a kind of self-empowerment of the human being, its "internal supremacy" as the authors put it. Against this background their concurrent evocation of a deterministic, biological sense of self-control and personal responsibility seems jarring (both, furthermore, were to be achieved through fairly strict discipline). Also jarring is the fact that Pearse and Scott Williamson often failed to make a clear distinction between their findings and their expectations of further insights. This is no doubt due partly to their book's purpose. One of its key goals was to attract donations and it articulates the dilemma involved in promising social relevance and innovative scientific findings while having to justify the need to spend a good deal of money generating them. Nonetheless, there is an explanatory gap here that cannot be put down solely to the pressure to acquire funds. It is hard to understand why Scott Williamson and Pearse, who had begun to work in a small, local welfare centre in the 1920s, took this work as the starting point for fundamental hypotheses about human development and society just a few years later. There is much evidence to suggest that this was bound up with a comparatively underdetermined concept of health. Perhaps the most honest definition in *The Case for Action* is: "Health is concerned with physiological balance or equilibrium, with the body's powers of reaction and with the development of latent powers. We do not yet know what this entails."[82]

What is clear is that a lot had happened between 1925 and 1931. For Pearse and Scott Williamson the focus had shifted from birth control and national efficiency to the functioning of life itself. And they were no longer solely concerned with practices of prevention but also with processes of intensification: they were eager to discover unknown potential inherent in life and allow it free rein. This required an approach quite different from the straightforward reformism that had motivated the original centre's wealthy West London initiators. Pearse and Scott Williamson saw themselves as scientists investigating human biological processes by conducting a social experiment. This threw up formidable epistemological problems centred on the researchers' above-mentioned self-image as knowledgeable friends, one they certainly maintained – and which soon required them to engage in a kind of participant observation. Scott Williamson's and Pearse's vision of themselves as technical assistants operating in the background of a collective mise en scène may, in fact, have been prescient when we consider the events that were to unfold in Peckham. Before explaining this in more detail I must briefly describe the stage on which these events occurred.

Notes

1 The Hon Mrs Ewen Montagu recollects the origins of the Pioneer Health Centre, 1998, WL, SA/PHC/B.1/1/1.
2 Notes re Pilot Scheme Plans, 1925, WL, SA/PHC/B.1/1/2, 2.
3 Ibid.
4 Ibid., 3, 2.
5 The Pioneer Health Centre at Peckham, September 24, 1934, TNA, MH 52/159.
6 Chairman's Report, November 24, 1925, WL, SA/PHC/A.1/1, 3–4.
7 Annual Report 1926, WL, SA/PHC/A.2/1, 4–5.
8 Ibid., 13.
9 Annual Report 1927, WL, SA/PHC/A.2/1, 5, 7, 9.
10 Speech to 2nd AGM of PHC, 1927, WL, SA/PHC/B.1/1/5, 5. Elsewhere we read: "We do not feel there will be very much danger of the men getting drunk. We think the very fact that they will be able to drink at leisure in the presence of their womenfolk in the homelike atmosphere prevailing in the Centre will prevent any such overindulgence." Secretary's Report for General Meeting, undated [c. 1927], WL, SA/PHC/A.1/1, 4.
11 Speech to 2nd AGM of PHC, 1927, WL, SA/PHC/B.1/1/5.
12 Chairman's Report, November 24, 1925, WL, SA/PHC/A.1/1, 6 (original emphasis).
13 Bill Luckin, "Revisiting the idea of degeneration in urban Britain, 1830–1900", *Urban History 33* (2006): 234–252. On the reality of the health status of the London population in the late 19th and early 20th centuries: Bill Luckin and Graham Mooney, "Urban history and historical epidemiology: The case of London, 1860–1920", *Urban History* 24 (1997): 37–55.
14 For the fundamentals, see: Anson Rabinbach, *The Human Motor. Energy, Fatigue, and the Origins of Modernity* (Berkeley: University of California Press, 1992). For an account of differences within Europe, see: Peter Baldwin, *Contagion and the State in Europe* (New York: Cambridge University Press, 2005).
15 Ministry of Health. Consultative Council on Medical and Allied Services. *Interim Report on the Future Provision of Medical and Allied Services 1920* (London: His Majesty's Stationery Office, 1920). The report also made a certain impact outside the United Kingdom: it inspired primary care and educational centres in New York and Ceylon. In 1931 the Rural Hygiene Conference of the League of Nations in Geneva also discussed health centres. The idea was put into practice on a grander scale in the USSR: Milton I. Roemer, *Evaluation of Community Health Centres* (Geneva: World Health Organization, 1972), 12–13. In Japan too there were state-run health centres, so-called "hokenjo", from 1937 onwards: Christopher Aldous and Akihito Suzuki, *Reforming Public Health in Occupied Japan, 1945–52: Alien Prescriptions?* (London, New York: Routledge, 2012), 163–176.
16 Jones, "Nothing Too Good for the People"; on the context, see John Stewart, *"The Battle for Health". A Political History of the Socialist Medical Association, 1930–51* (Aldershot: Ashgate, 1999), who also mentions later visits by SMA representatives to the second centre in Peckham: 52.

17 Hugh Cunningham, *The Children of the Poor. Representations of Childhood since the Seventeenth Century* (Oxford/Cambridge MA: Blackwell, 1991), 190–225.

18 On the scientization of research on poverty in the UK, see: Ian Gazeley, *Poverty in Britain, 1900–1965* (Basingstoke/London: Palgrave Macmillan, 2003).

19 Sally Alexander, "A New Civilization? London Surveyed 1928–1940s", *History Workshop* 65 (2007): 297–320.

20 See Ina Zweiniger-Bargielowska, *Managing the Body. Beauty, Health, and Fitness in Britain 1880–1939* (Oxford: Oxford University Press, 2010), 64–73, 151–153; Christopher Lawrence, "Regenerating England: An Introduction", in *Greater than the Parts: Holism in Biomedicine, 1920–1950*, ed. Christopher Lawrence and George Weisz (Oxford: Oxford University Press, 1998), 1–23.

21 Alysa Levene, "Between Less Eligibility and the NHS: The Changing Place of the Poor Law Hospitals in England and Wales, 1929–39", *Twentieth Century British History* 20 (2009): 322–345.

22 Steve Sturdy, "Hippocrates and the State Medicine: George Newman Outlines the Founding Policy of the Ministry of Health", in Lawrence and Weisz, *Greater than the Parts*, 112–134.

23 For an overview of the chequered history of British social medicine, see: Greta Jones, *Social Hygiene in Twentieth Century Britain* (London: Croom Helm, 1986); and Dorothy Porter, *Health, Civilisation and the State. A History of Public Health from Ancient to Modern Times* (London: Routledge, 1992); Steven Cherry, "Medicine and Public Health, 1900–1939", in *A Companion to Early Twentieth Century Britain*, ed. Christopher John Wrigley (Blackwell: Oxford, 2003), 405–423. For a more general account, see: Anne Hardy, *Health and Medicine in Britain since 1860* (Basingstoke: Palgrave Macmillan, 2001).

24 Zweiniger-Bargielowska, *Managing the Body*, 153–161.

25 Nigel Scotland, *Squires in the Slums: Settlements and Missions in Late-Victorian London* (London/New York: I.B. Tauris, 2007); Ruth Gilchrist and Tony Jeffs, eds., *Settlements, Social Change, and Community Action: Good Neighbours* (London/Philadelphia: Jessica Kingsley Publishers, 2001, several chapters of which mention the PHC). *Slumming* is likely to have played a role in these initiatives as well: Seth Koven, *Slumming, Sexual and Social Politics in Victorian London* (Princeton, NJ: Princeton University Press, 2004). As it happens, initially even the founders of the PHC regarded it as a settlement: Gerald Schlesinger, A Pioneer Health Centre, Peckham [late 1920s], WL, SA/PHC/B.1/5.

26 Karl H. Metz, "'Selbsthilfe'. Anmerkungen zu einer viktorianischen Idee". In *"Victorian Values". Arm und Reich im Viktorianischen England*, ed. Bernd Weisbrod (Bochum: Brockmeyer, 1987), 102. See also Stefan Collini, *Public Moralists. Political Thought and Intellectual Life in Britain 1850–1930* (Oxford: Oxford University Press, 1991).

27 Robert Humphreys, *Poor Relief and Charity 1869–1945. The London Charity Organization Society* (New York: Palgrave Macmillan, 2001).

28 Still worth reading on this process is: François Ewald, *L'état providence* (Paris: B. Grasset, 1986). But see also Harold Perkin, *The Rise of Professional Society. England since 1880* (London: Routledge, 1989); and Geoffrey Finlayson, *Citizen, State and Social Welfare in Britain 1830–1990* (Oxford: Clarendon Press, 1994).

29 See Patrick Joyce, *Democratic Subjects. The Self and the Social in Nineteenth-Century England* (Cambridge/New York: Cambridge University Press, 1994), 14–20.

30 *The Minority Report of the Poor Law Commission Part I. The Break-Up of the Poor Law. Ed. Sidney and Beatrice Webb* (Clifton: A.M. Kelley 1979), 549.

31 John Stewart, "'For a Healthy London': The Socialist Medical Association and the London County Council in the 1930s", *Medical History* 42 (1997): 417–443.

32 In what follows I will mostly refer to the two protagonists as Peckham *researchers*, a neutral description for two individuals, educated as doctors, who were – according

to their job description at the centre – initially its "medical officers", then its "medical directors", but soon saw themselves as "biologists", and even coined the neologism "bionomists": scientists who investigate the order of life (Pearse, *The Quality of Life*, 163). It was not just Pearse's and Scott Williamson's self-description that changed but also the way they referred to their research objects. From members of a health club, distinguished chiefly by their class affiliation, they turned into participants in a scientific experiment, human "guinea pigs". To remind us of their individual agency and the highly variable motives that led them to the centre, in most cases I will refer to them neutrally as its *users*.

33 On what follows, see esp. Mary Langman, G. S. W. and I. H. P. – approximate dates and places, 1983, WL, SA/PHC/C.13.

34 Reminiscences of St Mary's Road Peckham, June/October 1984, WL, SA/PHC/C.20.

35 Report of Speech at Nasmyth Club London, undated [c. 1937], WL, SA/PHC/D.2/4/3.

36 Jane Lewis and Barbara Brookes, "The Peckham Health Centre, 'PEP', and the Concept of General Practice during the 1930s and 1940s", *Medical History* 27 (1983): 158.

37 WL, SA/PHC/D.1/1, 2.

38 Pearse, *The Quality of Life*, 161–163.

39 Speech to Women's Advertising Club London, October 12, 1948, WL, SA/PHC/D.2/18/6.

40 This at least is how Frances Donaldson remembers things in her memoirs, the only published source on the private lives of those involved in the PHC: Frances Donaldson, *Child of the Twenties* (London: Rupert Hart-Davis 1959), 161, 163–164.

41 Tape 18: Mary Boast interviews Dr Innes Pearse, June 23, 1976, SLHA.

42 See Chapter 11.

43 Mary Langman, G. S. W. and I. H. P. – approximate dates and places, 1983, WL, SA/PHC/C.13.

44 Donaldson, *Child of the Twenties*, 162.

45 Reminiscences of St Mary's Road Peckham, 1984, WL, SA/PHC/C.20, 5.

46 Tape 18: Mary Boast interviews Dr Innes Pearse, June 23, 1976, SLHA.

47 Unknown sender to Henry Dale, December 18, 1928, TNA, FD 1/1023.

48 Henry Dale to Walter Morley Fletcher, November 19, 1929, TNA, FD 1/1023.

49 Illegible to Fletcher, January 30, 1932, TNA, FD 1/1023.

50 Fletcher to Pearse, April 27, 1932, TNA, FD 1/1023.

51 John Stewart, "The Political Economy of the British National Health Service, 1945–1975: Opportunities and Constraints?", *Medical History* 52 (2008): 455.

52 Speech to the League of Nations Union, undated [1929], WL, SA/PHC/B.1/1/8, 1 f.

53 Paper on Scientific Enquiry into Social Disintegration, undated [c. 1931], WL, SA/PHC/B.1/1/6.

54 Untitled speech manuscript, 1929, WL, SA/PHC/B.2/1, 3 f.

55 Scott Williamson to Pilgrim Trust, January 1931, WL, SA/PHC/B.2/2.

56 See for example the Ministry of Health's appraisal: The Pioneer Health Centre at Peckham, September 24, 1934, TNA, MH 52/159.

57 Financing PHC, undated [1929], WL, SA/PHC/B.2/1.

58 GSW (Finance), undated [1929], WL, SA/PHC/B.2/1.

59 Memorandum and Articles of Association, February 26, 1931, LMA, LCC/PH/PHS/1/7.

60 The vanity inherent in the philanthropy of this period is evident in the fact that donors might hope to see their own names in these brochures alongside those of the centre's illustrious patrons. These included an array of earls, counts, viscounts and lords as well as the bishop of Salisbury. Reference was also made to the PHC's scientific advisory committee. In the early 1930s this consisted of a number of

professors, including Julian Huxley, but also the presidents of the Royal Society and British Dental Association.

61 Circular from Sainsbury [early 1930s], WL, SA/PHC/B.2/5.
62 The Health of the Race – A new Plan of National Health-Building – Its Vital Importance to every Taxpayer, undated [c. 1933], WL, SA/PHC/B.2/11/10.
63 The Crisis [early 1930s], WL, SA/PHC/B.2/11/7.
64 Scott Williamson and Pearse, *The Case for Action*, 124, 132.
65 SA/PHC/B.1/4.
66 Scott Williamson and Pearse, *The Case for Action*, v–vii, vii.
67 Ibid., 117, 4, 6, 39, 42, 44.
68 Ibid., 7. The findings of these examinations make up only a small portion of the book. Information on the prevalence of specific diseases can be found in the (sparse) endnotes.
69 Ibid., 9–10.
70 Ibid., 15, 86.
71 Ibid., 38, 47, 53, 55.
72 Ibid., 65. For Scott Williamson and Pearse, ideally this natural unit already began to take shape through one's choice of partner, which guaranteed the greatest possible "chemical" complementarity of man and woman as "organs", with the woman "sensing" the right partner. Interestingly, they had no objection to women's efforts to achieve independence, which seemed to make a biologically successful choice of partner possible in the first place (ibid., 73). Against this background it comes as no surprise that Pearse and Scott Williamson were not in favour of genetic interventionism. They certainly deployed eugenic arguments – highlighting, for example, what they regarded as the absurdity that the English were world-class horse-breeders yet knew nothing of the potential to improve the quality of human beings. But they believed that most qualities worthy of promotion could be more effectively elicited by interpersonal stimulation. They conceived of intelligence, for example, as a mental "adaptability" that could be trained through stimulation emanating from the social environment. See Innes H. Pearse, "Racial Culture", *Journal of State Medicine* 44, no. 10 (1927): 1–69.
73 Scott Williamson and Pearse, *The Case for Action*, 69.
74 Ibid., 120.
75 Ibid., 121, 39, 127.
76 Ibid., 129–130.
77 Ibid., 144.
78 Ibid., 152–153 (original emphasis).
79 Ibid., 102, 135.
80 Ibid., 136.
81 Ibid., 137.
82 Ibid., 111.

3 St Mary's Road, S.E.15

New premises, initial routines? (1931–1935)

By 1931, when *The Case for Action* was published, architect Ernest Brander Musman had already drawn up a blueprint for a new building on St Mary's Road; an image of it even took up a whole page of the book (Figure 3.1). A number of surviving sketches show that Musman's proposed ground plan was quite different from the open design of the completed building.[1] His outlines comprise clearly separated rooms that create equally distinct spheres for the centre's users on the one hand and directors on the other. The building featured an imposing oval entrance hall, yet members were expected to use separate side entrances. The first floor was dominated by a large meeting room for the centre's directors, flanked by two offices and a staff apartment. Glass played no significant role in the building's interior.

The collaboration with Musman, however, was discontinued before the year was out; apparently his plan was too expensive. Pearse and Scott Williamson set out to find someone to help them create a graphic aid to communication with other architects, with the Architectural Association School of Architecture (AA) recommending architecture student J.M. Richards.[2] In the autumn of 1933 they then engaged Sir E. Owen Williams, with whom John Sainsbury had come into contact during the renovation of the Boots plant in Nottingham. The Management Committee had sent Richards's sketches to five architects, including Williams, to ascertain whether such a building could be constructed for £25,000.[3] This unconventional approach, which bypassed the need for an official call for bids and costly preliminary designs, provoked sharp criticism from one of the architects contacted, Harry Goodhart-Rendel, who went so far as to inform the relevant professional association, the Royal Institute of British Architects (RIBA). Williams was apparently chosen in part because he was formally a civil engineer and as such immune to censure by RIBA.[4] Above all, though, his cost estimate of £22,500 managed to stay below the available sum.[5]

Williams may have taken Richards's sketches as his starting point. But in contrast to the two directors' retrospective accounts, there is no indication in the planning-related documents that the researchers and architect worked together on the ground plan.[6] This is not an insignificant point: many of the above-mentioned studies in architectural history analyse the building as the

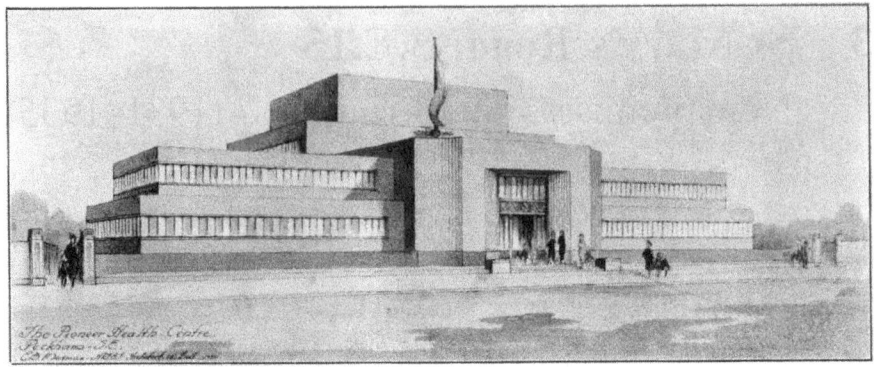

Figure 3.1 E.M. Musman's proposal of 1931 – a monumental building, featuring
        expressionist details (the zigzag frieze above the portal) and modernist
        elements, such as the continuous ribbon windows. The perspective chosen,
        with the observer looking up at the property, underlines the impression of
        a hierarchical sequence of spaces, as do the staircase-like tiering of the
        floors and the emphatic axial symmetry. Probably for want of relevant
        templates, Musman made the building look much like a government
        agency or public institution, including a flagpole and small outside
        staircase.
(George Scott Williamson and Innes H. Pearse, *The Case for Action. A Survey of
Everyday Life under Modern Industrial Conditions, with Special Reference to the
Question of Health*. London: Faber & Faber, 1931, inside cover)

central element in a consciously conceived social experiment.[7] There is little
evidence to suggest, however, that the building was a direct expression of the
demands the doctors made of it as a social laboratory.

Observation platforms and niches for congregation

In the spring of 1935, after a comparatively brief construction period, the
building was ready for occupation. Set back from the street by a few metres, it
stood empty on a tree-fringed plot (Figure 3.2). Plain as it was, it might have
been mistaken for an industrial structure with its rectangular ground plan and
flat roof. Only the glass facade on the first and second floors, leavened by
roughly semi-circular protrusions – small bays with subtly overhanging
ledges – suggested a different purpose. This glass facade was flanked by two
avants-corps. Rough squares, like most of the window panes, these lent the
building a recumbent, horizontal air. The sides of the building were even
more austere, with the precast concrete skeleton clearly discernible. Above all,
the building seemed prosaic because, in sharp contrast to Musman's plan, it
lacked a central portal. Certainly, the windows on the street-side ground floor
were slightly set back into the brickwork; but the main entrances and the
narrow staircases were located at the building's rear corners. Here the building's core was indented somewhat from the first floor upwards, allowing for a

large balcony. The facade was plastered in white, while the banisters, gutters and numerous door and window frames were finished in a darkened varnish, a striking subject for black and white photographs.[8]

Inside, the centre was subdivided roughly into three functional zones (Figures 3.3, 3.4). The ground floor was devoted to physical activities. It housed showers, changing rooms and toilets and a small swimming pool for children, which could be accessed directly from the nursery. This was situated behind the set-back street-side facade, which could be opened up as needed, allowing the children to play in the open air. The ground floor also housed the machine room for the (novel) electrical heating, water tanks, the water filtration system and store rooms. Also on ground level were the gymnasium, which took up two floors, and, on the opposite side of the building, a large room with a stage. Initially referred to as a lecture hall and later as a theatre, this was the site of concerts and other performances but also sporting activities such as badminton. The first floor was ascribed a social function. Its rear side featured a self-service cafeteria and kitchen while at the front there was a large lounge, the scene of dance nights and Christmas and New Year parties. Finally, the second floor was the medical zone. This accommodated the laboratories and consulting rooms and a further two rooms for dental treatment, later evidently used for other purposes such as band practice. On the wings of this floor other rooms were designated for study and recreation, while the front side was reserved for the library. The building was crowned by an asphalt roof terrace with a glazed gable at its centre.

At the heart of the building was a large swimming pool. The second largest in London at the time of its construction, it was built to Olympic standards,

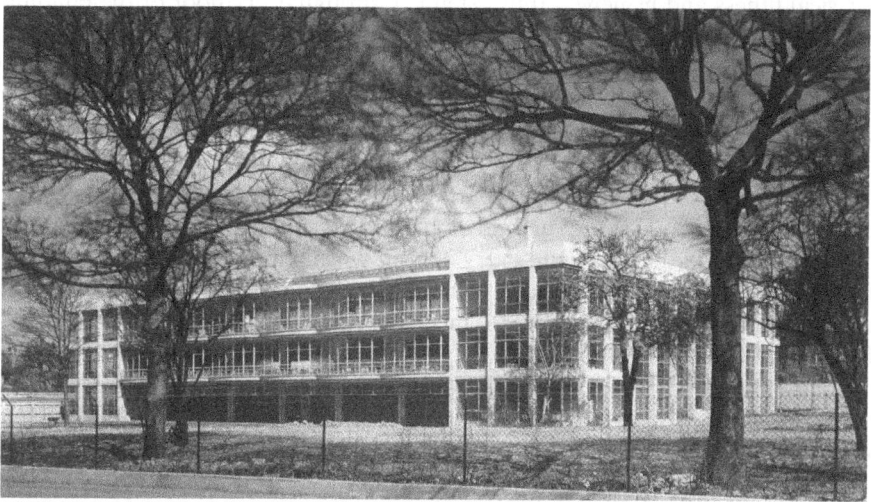

Figure 3.2 The Pioneer Health Centre shortly before it opened in 1935, viewed from St Mary's Road (Pioneer Health Centre, Peckham, St Mary's Road, Peckham, London, Dell & Wainwright/RIBA Library Photographs Collection)

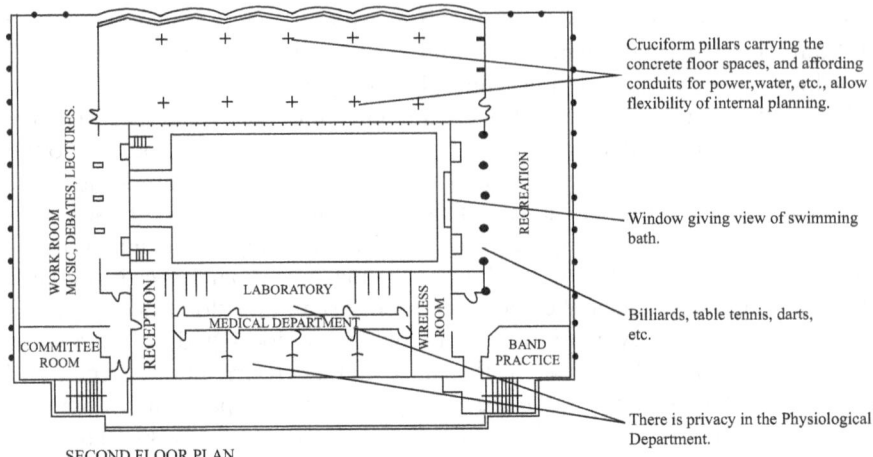

SECOND FLOOR PLAN

Figure 3.3 Plan of the second floor with annotations concerning, for example, the view
of the swimming pool
(Redrawn from: Innes H. Pearse and Lucy H. Crocker, *The Peckham Experiment. A Study
of the* Living *Structure of Society.* London: Allen & Unwin, 1943, 300, image detail)

as was the concrete diving platform. At water level the pool was separated
from the lounge and cafeteria by glazed interior walls, with access through two
small doors. The main access route for bathers, however, was provided by two
interior staircases, leading from the changing rooms on the ground floor to just
short of the pool's edge. The large space containing the pool – a symbol of
physical fitness and hygiene – thus extended through every floor of the building.

Clearly, then, the different spheres (social, physical, and medical) overlapped.
There was no radical functional division as propagated by many advocates of
modernism at the time, to whom the building's axial symmetry would have
appeared rather conventional, even redundant: two rooms for dental treatment,
two entrances, two staircases. The mirroring of the building's two halves did, however, correspond to the division of genders to some degree. There were two separate
circulatory pathways on the ground floor, with its changing rooms, and in the
medical zone, in other words in every area in which clothing might be removed.
Initially, even the medical section itself was divided into two spheres by a swing
door, featuring separate entrances for men and women on each side of the hallway.
In addition a number of doors on the second floor were painted red to indicate
restricted access. The spaces reserved for user activities here were also designated
for gender-specific activities, with an area for the women's textile work and a
workshop for the men.

That said, there were very few closed doors in the centre. Photographs taken
shortly before it was opened show rooms that, while not necessarily large, are light;
above all, they reveal a building in which the transitions between rooms are rather
subtle.[9] For instance, one could circumvent the swimming pool in its entirety but it
remained visible from two sides thanks to the glass dividing walls (Figure 3.4). At

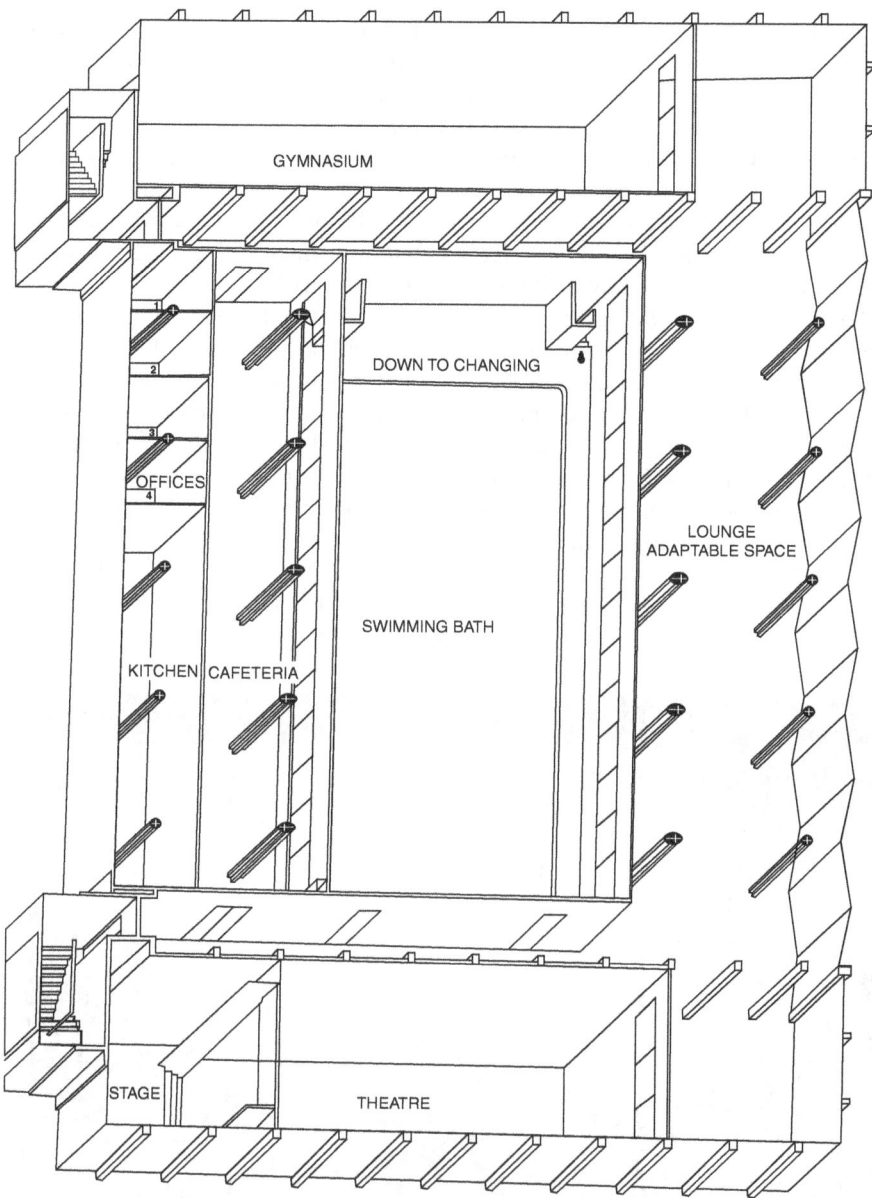

Figure 3.4 Axonometric section at second floor height. Clearly visible are the central
swimming bath and the numerous glass apertures within the building
(Redrawn from: George Scott Williamson and Innes H. Pearse, *Biologists in Search of
Material. An Interim Report on the Work of the Pioneer Health Centre, Peckham.*
London: Faber & Faber, 1938, without page number)

several points visual axes penetrated the entire depth of the building. Veritable viewing platforms were created on the first floor, where a panoramic window provided views of the gymnasium, and on the first floor, where viewers could observe what was happening in the swimming pool (Figure 3.5).

Openness was facilitated by an innovative construction, whose key elements were cruciform reinforced concrete columns placed at regular intervals and broadening out near the roof. On the street side these columns were set back from the glass front, creating space for window niches. The interior walls' brickwork consisted chiefly of lightweight breeze blocks.

The centre's furniture and fittings were also novel. The crockery in the cafeteria was of damage-resistant aluminium. Cork flooring contributed to the homey atmosphere by reflecting the ceiling lights with a warm orange glow. On the "social" floor there were crates with glass windows containing toys and sports equipment; castors allowed them to be moved around freely.[10] They were designed by interior architect Christopher Nicholson, who also contributed installations such as the changing rooms and shower cubicles, and a number of tables and chairs, many of them of tubular steel. These were not only cheap to make but stackable and thus well-suited to multipurpose rooms.[11] The same went for the V-shaped wooden table modules, which could be fitted together to create a circle or elongated tables (Figure 3.6). This design seems to have been

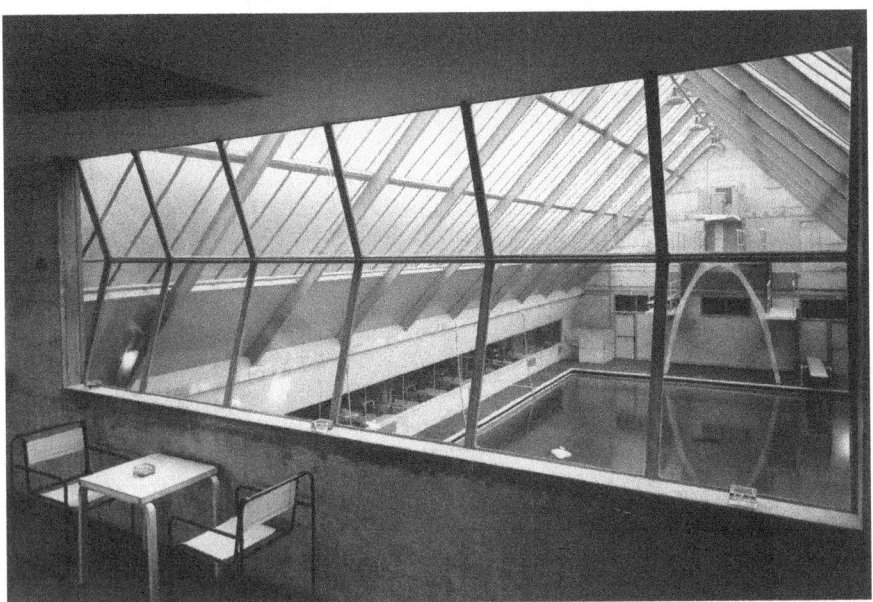

Figure 3.5 View of the swimming pool from the medical section – diving platform at back right, glass roof at the top, cafeteria to the left next to the pool
(Pioneer Health Centre, St Mary's Road, Peckham, London: view of the swimming pool from one of the recreation rooms, Dell & Wainwright/RIBA Library Photographs Collection)

rooted in the hope that a variety of social constellations would crystallize spontaneously at the centre.[12]

It was this hope that also emanated from J.M. Richards's euphoric 1935 article in the *Architectural Review* on the new building he had helped design. He welcomed the fact that the areas of circulation adhered closely to those zones in which "self-determination" was undesirable, such as the edge of the pool or the narrow staircases. He considered the latter particularly well-conceived as they discouraged loitering. Above all, though, he praised the street-front bays because they promised to foster the formation of social groups:

> [S]hallow bays […] encourage natural congregation into groups; but they are not sufficiently pronounced to invite marked separation into cliques. [The] semi-privacy of the bays along either side preserves the feeling of stability necessary to counteract the restlessness a mobile population would tend to induce.[13]

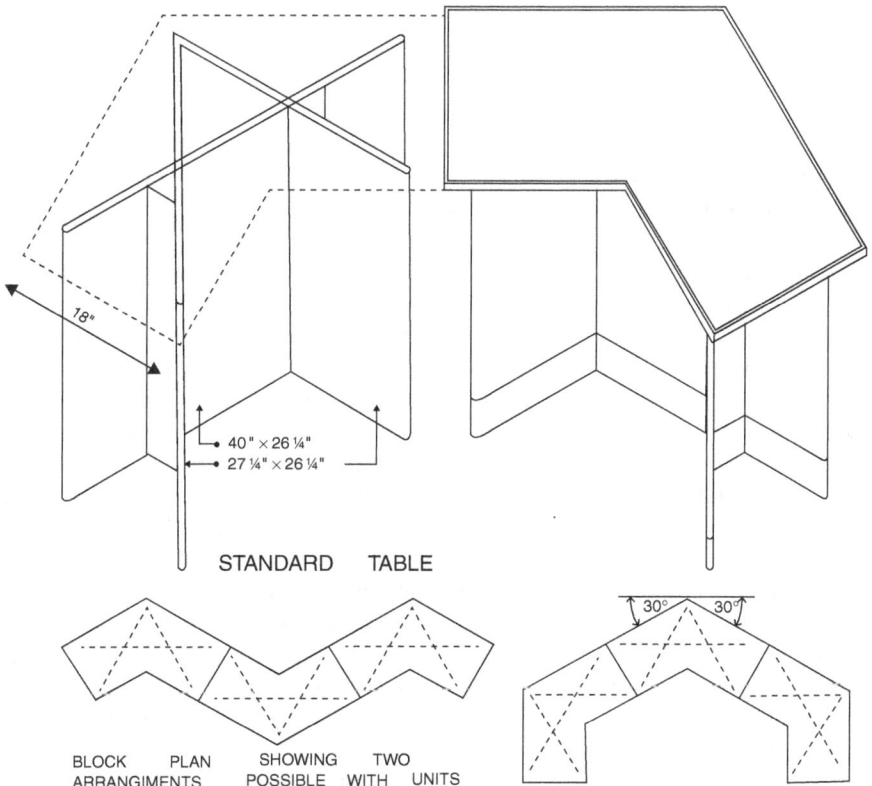

Figure 3.6 Nicholson's modular standard table for the centre. At bottom two possible combinations
(Redrawn from: J.M. Richards, "The Idea Behind the Idea", *The Architectural Review* 7(1935): 210, image detail)

So for Richards, soon to become one of Britain's most influential architectural critics, the building was designed to foster certain types of collective behaviour within its walls while impeding others. Its ground plan seemed to create a balanced relationship between "natural" social dynamism and stability, while preventing isolation and unproductive passivity.

Success stories

On April 29, 1935, more than five years after its predecessor's closure, all forms of official approval had been obtained and the new building could open. It had already been presented to journalists in March, apparently in the presence of around 1,000 individuals.[14] Scott Williamson gave an enthusiastic speech to mark the occasion. The centre, he asserted, would provide an answer to fundamental contemporary questions, an answer consonant with the English national character: "The English way is that of persuasion and education of a free and responsible people."[15] By December 1935 Pearse and Scott Williamson could proudly announce that within just a few months the centre had managed to attract 350 families as regular users, despite having rejected around 100 membership applications (because the applicants did not live in Peckham), and despite the fact that many users had soon stopped coming (centre staff put this down to the high house-moving rate in the district and the centre's novelty). Earlier, invitations dropped through letter boxes on every street within walking distance of the centre had advertised the project to potential members (Figure 3.7).[16]

The first 12 months, according to the annual report of 1936, saw a vast number of initial examinations – 4,500 in total. These were carried out by up to four doctors, a biochemist and a laboratory assistant, working virtually round the clock, and they were surprisingly popular. This high figure is telling when set against the centre's membership, which had barely grown. It is a first indication of the fact which would trouble the centre for most of its existence, that plenty of Peckham residents were interested in the cheap preventive check-up, without needing to be talked into it – and without wanting to become permanent club members. Nonetheless, the annual report announced that a genuine community had already come into being. For example, there had been a number of parties, and members generally displayed a conspicuous "hunger for social life".[17] A number of surviving programmes do in fact show that users were engaging in a wide range of leisure activities shortly after the centre opened. They could attend so-called keep-fit classes; they could swim, play badminton, table tennis or water polo, box and even fence. There were concerts, tea dances and cards nights. The year 1936 saw the establishment of a theatre group and an arts-and-crafts club for children.[18] These activities cost between one penny (half an hour of darts) and sixpence (billiards), but they were free for children under 16. Each family had to renew its membership on a weekly basis by paying one shilling.[19] The payment of this contribution – which apparently most Peckham households could manage but which was far from trivial[20] – was noted on the membership cards given to each family member, to whom the building was open daily from 2pm to 10.30pm.

STREETS IN THE DISTRICT.

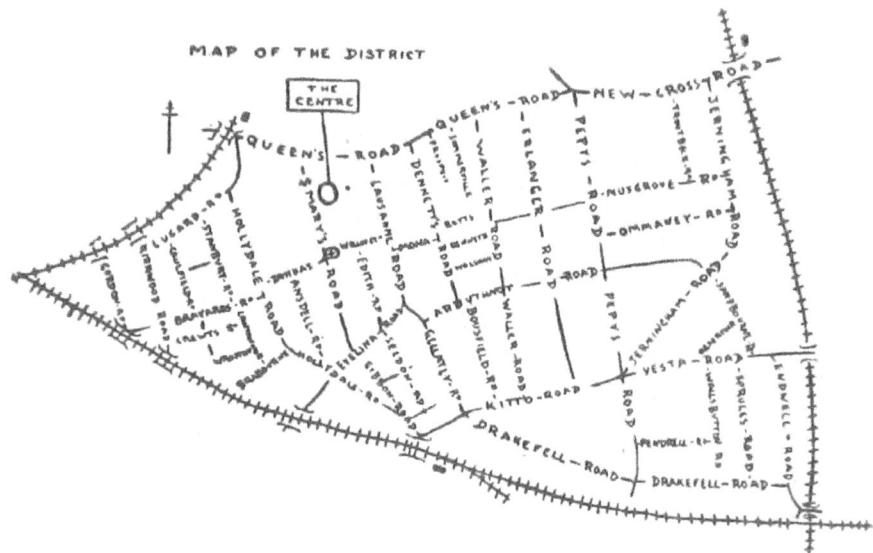

Figure 3.7 The centre's catchment area in the mid 1930s
(The Centre, St Mary's Road, Peckham, SE15, undated [c. 1937], WL, SA/PHC/B.3/22/1)

Evidently, specific rhythms of usage soon took hold. In the early afternoon it was chiefly housewives with small children who visited the centre – the nursery, which was open until evening, admitted children of up to five years of age. When school finished, around 4pm, the schoolchildren arrived; in the 1930s 200–300 of them attended the centre daily. The gym was reserved for them until 7pm, and they could also make use of roller skates, trampolines, board games and the library, which mainly contained works of fiction and children's books. Towards evening the men arrived, and the activities within the centre shifted to dancing, card games and the after-work beer in the self-service cafeteria – this at least is the harmonious picture painted by the annual reports. From 1936 on these also emphasized that all activities were self-administered, for example with respect to the allocation of rooms.[21]

Other sources, however, suggest that social life within the centre was less conflict-free than implied in the official reports. In fact initially it was plagued by vandalism. The unexpectedly slow rate of recruitment of new users, moreover, was a serious economic problem for the centre's operators. But before turning to these difficulties I would like to jump forward in time. It is well worth taking a close look at the researchers' most important book, *The Peckham Experiment. A Study of the Living Structure of Society* (their emphasis), published in 1943 by Allen and Unwin, a firm that published many books by influential natural scientists at the time. This reveals just how much the directors' interpretations had changed by 1939, when the war triggered the new centre's closure and Pearse began to write about the insights gained from it. For this shift has much to do with events in the centre shortly after it opened, which I will reconstruct in detail later on.

Notes

1 London (Southwark): Pioneer Health Centre, Saint Mary's Road, Peckham, competition designs, undated [c. 1930], RIBA, PA354/9(1–20).
2 Richards later described their collaboration as follows: "All I had to do was make notes of the sizes of the spaces they wanted to provide [...] and draw these out to help the doctors investigate further how one space should relate to another and what there would be room for at each level of the site." J.M. Richards, *Memoirs of an Unjust Fella* (London: Weidenfeld and Nicolson, 1980), 88.
3 Minutes, Board of Management/Management Committee, October 26, 1933, WL, SA/PHC/A.1/3. One of the candidates was Wells Coates, who was constructing the famous Isokon Building in Hampstead, London, at the time.
4 Goodhart-Rendel to Ian MacAlister, October 24, 1933, RIBA, Harry Stuart Goodhart-Rendel, Greh/3/1.
5 Minutes, Board of Management/Management Committee, November 2, 1933, WL, SA/PHC/A.1/3.
6 Surviving plans in Williams's literary estate feature only negligible revisions (Design for the Pioneer Health Centre, Saint Mary's Road, Peckham, Williams, Sir Evan Owen, 1890–1969, RIBA, DR52/7). The key concerns raised by the Management Committee when it examined these plans concerned aspects such as window-cleaning and heating costs: Minutes, Board of Management/Management Committee, February 1, 1934, WL, SA/PHC/A.1/3.
7 This is most apparent in Kozlovsky, *The Architectures of Childhood*, ch. 1. In contrast, David Cottam, author of a history of Williams's work, argues that the ground plan and even the finished building's modernist outward appearance were the result of cost considerations and thus Williams's engineering logic. See: "Pioneer Health Centre", in *Sir Owen Williams 1890–1969*, ed. David Cottam (London: Architectural Association Publications, 1986), 99.
8 Such photographs were soon published along with night-time views of the centre that reverse the light-dark contrast. In these photographs light emanates from the many windows; the building's inner life seems to radiate into its surroundings, the evening facade becoming a projection screen for the activities within. The silhouettes of dancing figures, for example, were thus displayed on the building's exterior, as the Peckham researchers themselves noted. This, they asserted, aroused the curiosity of some passers-by: Pearse and Crocker, *The Peckham Experiment*, 71.
9 "Pioneer Health Centre, Peckham", *The Architectural Review* 77 (1935): 209–216. The photos by M.O. Dell and H.L. Wainwright are little works of art, some of them taken from oblique angles that effectively underscore the abstract lines and seriality of the shower rooms or ceiling construction.
10 Pearse and Crocker, *The Peckham Experiment*, 198.
11 G. Summer, "Plywood Furniture at the Pioneer Health Centre", *design for today* 3 (1935): 219.
12 Designs & working drawings for offices, cubicles, kitchen & furniture for the Pioneer Health Centre, Saint Mary's Road, Southwark, London, by Christopher Nicholson. RIBA, PA1206/4(1–58).
13 J.M. Richards, "The Idea Behind the Idea", *The Architectural Review* 77 (1935): 207–209; see also J.M. Richards, "Pioneer Work at Peckham", *The Architect's Journal* 81 (1935): 509. Shortly afterwards Richards also discussed the Finsbury Health Centre, mentioned at the start of the book, which he was less enthusiastic about: "Finsbury Makes a Programme", *The Architectural Review* 85 (1939): 9.

14 Annual Report 1935, WL, SA/PHC/A.2. See also the reports in the *Daily Herald*, April 29, 1935; *Daily Mirror*, March 3, 1935; *Manchester Guardian*, February 14, 1933; *New Statesman*, March 3, 1935; *Observer*, March 1, 1935; and in the *Illustrated London News*, April 6, 1935. The project on the Queen's Road, meanwhile, had remained below the radar of the print media, and *The Case for Action* had attracted only a few, albeit favourable, reviews: Mary B. Gilson, "Health a Family Problem", *Survey* (1931): 660; "The Case for Action", *Review of Biology* 1, no. 1 (1932).
15 Untitled speech manuscript, 1935, WL, SA/PHC/B.3/1, 2–3.
16 First eight months. May–Dec. 1935, WL, SA/PHC/B.3/8/1.
17 Annual Report 1936, WL, SA/PHC/A.2, 6, 10.
18 Programme for Coronation Week, May 1936, WL, SA/PHC/B.3/2.
19 Pearse and Crocker, *The Peckham Experiment*, 72, 303–304.
20 According to Ian Gazeley, for example, in 1935 skilled workers in the British textile industry earned an average gross wage of 49.2 shillings (men) and 27.5 shillings (women): Gazeley, *Poverty in Britain*, 69.
21 Annual Report 1936, WL, SA/PHC/A.2, 11.

4 *"Living* structure of society"
The magnum opus and its scientific context

Innes Pearse wrote *The Peckham Experiment* in close collaboration with her assistant Lucy Crocker, their work financed by writing scholarships from the Halley Stewart Trust, an influential foundation within the British medical research landscape.[1] Their objectives are not really clear from the text itself. Evidently they advocated the establishment of more centres of the Peckham type – while the preface at least, addressed to the "intelligent layman", indicates that otherwise nothing less than the end of civilization is at stake.[2] Pearse and Crocker, however, had very little practical advice to offer on how to avert this catastrophe. Instead they appear to have regarded the book – to a greater degree than *The Case for Action* – as a contribution to basic research, as evident in a short passage right at the start on the centre's prehistory. Gaining a better understanding of human nature was already the priority in 1926, the authors assert here. Furthermore, they had been eager to establish a more precise definition of health: in contrast to the perspective generally prevalent within conventional medicine, they had attempted to understand it not just as the absence of illness but as *positivity*.[3] But against this background the publication's subheading is rather striking: *"living* structure of society." Despite the italics, this implied a work of social science rather than medical research.

We need only flick through the book to be struck by a so-called Chapter in Photographs (which I will be looking at in more detail in Chapter 6), and a table on the front cover. I will already mention here that for many readers the latter represented the essence of the experiment. Under the caption "The Burden of Disorder", it visualizes the alarming results of the initial examination of 1,206 families (Figure 4.1). Differentiated by age, two bar charts, one for the men, one for the women, contrast the absolute number of users among whom disorders were diagnosed with those free of abnormalities. There are also two area charts illustrating the breakdown of the two groups in percentage terms: just 4% of the almost 2,000 female members examined, for example, were free of symptoms of ill health.[4]

A number of appendices make a similarly no-nonsense impression. Here we find a table with information on users' ocular, blood and urine values, height and weight. Also shown are a diagnostic questionnaire for use in the laboratory

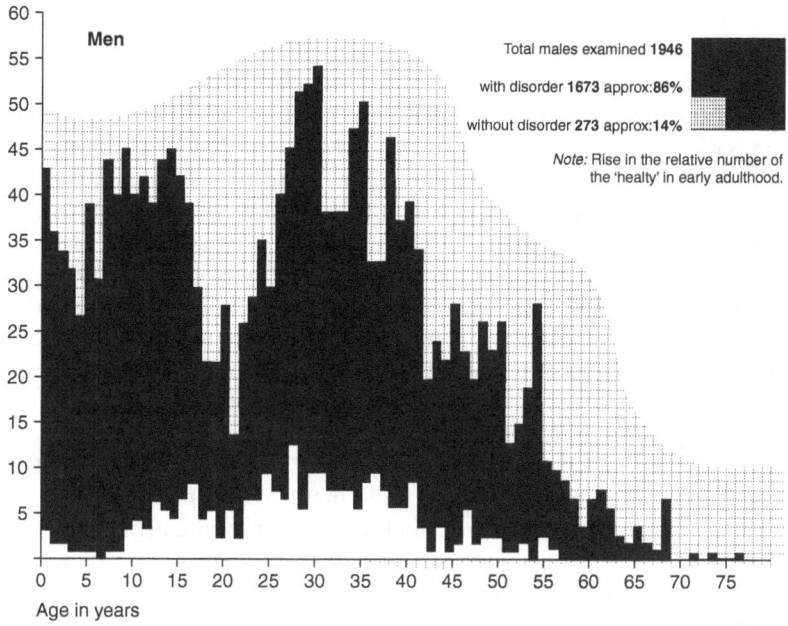

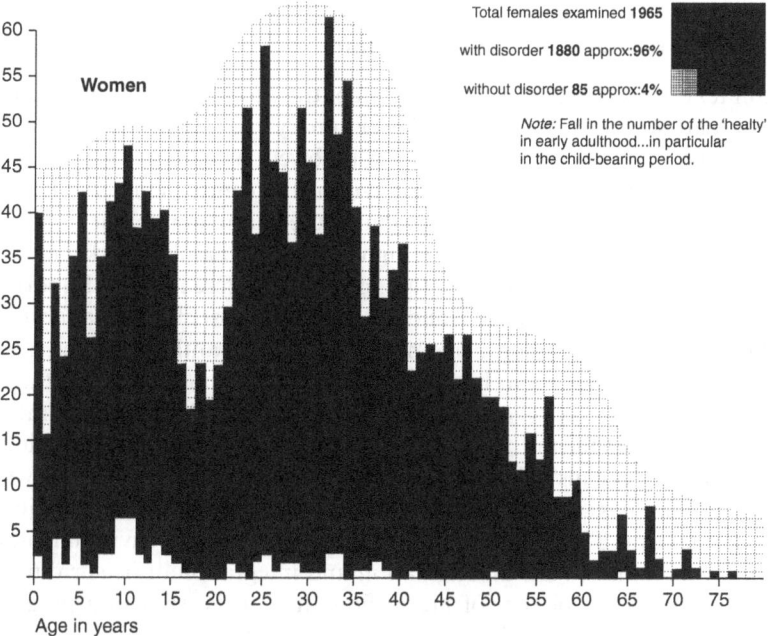

Figure 4.1 "The Burden of Disorder"
(Redrawn from: Innes H. Pearse and Lucy H. Crocker, *The Peckham Experiment. A Study of the* Living *Structure of Society.* London: Allen & Unwin, 1943, inside cover)

and several so-called tonoscillogrammes – the results of a novel method of measuring blood pressure. Certain findings of the medical examination – for example on users' iron deficiency and worm infestations – are listed separately. The costs of the medical work are itemized in tabular form; the centre's financial situation is discussed; the building is described with the help of the ground plans for all three floors; the activities on offer in the centre are listed; and the average number of visitors is mentioned according to days of the week and time of day.

Finally, the appendix includes a table itemizing the occupations of the adult members of the 500 member families. This is the only place in the book to provide more detail on the socioeconomic conditions in the area. As indicated earlier, craftsmen, white-collar workers and skilled labourers were in the majority (among the men). The largest occupational group consisted of workers in the engineering industry (100 individuals) and transportation (89). The most common occupations were "unclassified clerks" (50 men, 10 women), shop assistants (26 men, 20 women), mechanics (25 men, 1 woman), electricians (16 men), typists (15 women), bus drivers (12 men), and printers (10 men). There were 8 police sergeants, 8 postmen, 2 doctors, 2 bakers and 2 artists, 1 student, 1 private detective, while one woman stated her occupation as "paper flower maker". Some 432 female members evidently described themselves as housewives, while just over half the working members indicated that they were permanently employed.[5]

The social environment as growth medium

The main text of the book stands in sharp contrast to these add-ons. It consists of three broad sections. A number of preliminary theoretical remarks and an account of the PHC's modus operandi are followed, as in *The Case for Action*, by a description of a reproductive cycle within the centre. This is followed by sections dedicated to the social integration of the centre community.

Life, to quote Pearse and Crocker's highly abstract initial remarks, manifests itself as a "function" of its own perpetual process of differentiation. Importantly, the "unit" of life within which this function becomes most clearly manifest is not the individual. Thus, in biology, one must observe the anthill, not the ant; the hive rather than the individual bee. The same goes for human beings: the basic biological unit of all social organization is the family. Men and women are physiologically different and must therefore be understood as cooperating but "diverse parts or organs of a unified organism". The human being will be healthy if he complies with this functional law, which governs more than just the couple-as-organism. The latter operates in synthesis with its environment, concurrently contributing to the differentiation and integration of its surroundings: "This is the functional picture of life in flow. It is to be seen in a progressive mutual synthesis participated in by both organism and environment. It is wholeness – Health."[6]

Informed by this holistic thinking, which even by the standards of the day seems profoundly moulded by the idea of gender difference (and gender complementarity), the authors come to a radical conclusion. The individual is significant solely as an element in a "progressive order". Pearse and Crocker, in fact, liken the idea of the autonomous individual to the cancerous cell with its isolated, dysfunctional growth. "Can it then be that Man is himself but a cell in the body of Cosmos ...", they write, tellingly omitting a question mark. What wise men have long suspected, the centre may soon be able to prove: the existence of an "all pervading order: Nature".[7]

By now, then, the Peckham Experiment was permeated by a vitalism that had little in common with the parental advisory service founded just over 15 years earlier. Pearse and Crocker believed themselves to be hot on the heels of life itself – though the meaning of the term "life" in their book overlaps greatly with that of "Health" (generally with a capital letter, like a deity), "nature" and "function". In fact *The Peckham Experiment* displays a general tendency for overlapping lexical fields, logical leaps and a conceptual framework even more idiosyncratic than that found in *The Case for Action*. The researchers believed they had identified a universally valid developmental law, which they typically conveyed through the term "nurture". Its broad array of associations (nutrition, enrichment, care, fostering, even education) allowed semantic jumps from concrete physiological nourishment to communication and social processes, such as learning from others. For Pearse and Crocker, then, every conceivable form of interaction could be interpreted as subprocesses of the same growth process, whether this meant biochemical reactions or friendships between families. This is evident in their interpretation of embryonic development, which they use to undergird their thesis. The differentiation of the embryonic cells, the authors tell us, is a result of the exchange of "material" between sperm and egg cell, fertilized egg cell and womb. And this process of exchange must be understood – with a social metaphor slipping in here – as mutual "familiarisation".[8]

Unfortunately, according to Pearse and Crocker, physiological laboratory work is ill suited to the investigation of such processes. In fact it distorts reality by isolating discrete chemical processes rather than observing their interactions as a whole. In Peckham, therefore, the researchers had created an entirely novel experiment: a situation that fostered syntheses between individuals. They had been able to study families in their "natural habitat" with a "sturdy sample of society" at hand. Though the authors make no comment on the fact, the working classes of the 1920s had thus become representatives of the British population as a whole – "good swimmers in midstream", as they write.[9] Bound up with this, the validity of their ideas extends beyond a specific social milieu to the human species as a whole.

This explains why the authors set out their biological ideas before providing a description of the actual workings of the centre. Pearse and Crocker present the latter as a natural growth medium that has increasingly been enriched with stimulants – a social "placenta" as they put it elsewhere in the text. They view the centre as an accumulator of information that users can, so to speak, soak up and "digest" in line with their proclivities and abilities. The building, they contend, was consciously designed as a diffusor of knowledge and as a space for testing it out. Its transparent, contact-facilitating architectural structure was also chosen for this purpose. Even the principle of self-service in operation in the cafeteria, the authors claim, was based on factors other than mere cost or efficiency: it was intended to light an initial, activating spark while simultaneously prompting consideration for others.[10]

But it was above all the conversations with the doctors, which Pearse and Crocker describe in detail, that were meant to trigger new behaviours. Families interested in the centre were given a tour through the house, ending in one of the doctors' waiting rooms. Here they were given an enrolment talk informing them of the centre's modus operandi and objectives. Afterwards the family could decide whether or not to take up membership and make individual appointments for medical examinations. Over the next few weeks family members were examined individually, men by male doctors, women and children by female ones. Families then attended the family consultation together. Deliberately informal, this meeting took place with both doctors in attendance. They began by reporting their findings on the children's state of health, who were then instructed to leave the room. Then it was the parents' turn, first the man, then the woman. More intimate matters were discussed, such as contraception and family planning. Almost all the family members' examination results, then, were discussed collectively, with the doctors emphasizing that it was up to the families themselves whether, and if so how, to respond to any problems that may have been detected. According to the authors both the medical diagnosis and information on the various options open to users were thus deliberately fed into their social environment. In any case, we learn, following these conversations many families had begun to contemplate what they had in common, their shared secrets and desires – a touching fact. But the consultations, the book asserts, also gave the doctors the opportunity to get to know the family as a whole, to identify behavioural patterns and social conflicts conducive to illness. For example, they closely observed family members' reactions to the results of the examinations, which often seemed to articulate unhealthy intra-familial frictions.[11]

Overall, Pearse and Crocker tell us, the examinations revealed that more than 90% of the individuals examined were sick in one way or another. This, they assert, represents a major problem for the British economy, but one that can be solved through a national early diagnosis programme. More interesting from a scientific point of view, the authors contend, is the unexpectedly high number of undiagnosed diseases and, above all, ones of which those afflicted were unaware. They explain that, in light of this observation, they have decided to distinguish more sharply between "disorder" and "disease", or between "well-being" and "health": a literal "dis-ease", that is, a clearly evident dysfunction, prompts a visit to the doctor; but the "dis-order" is the gravest problem because it is antecedent. For the authors, then, the term disorder encompasses not just physical problems such as infections but also disease-causing social phenomena, such as an unnoticed vitamin deficiency resulting from a family's faulty nutritional habits. However, disorders, our authors point out, can trigger remarkable compensatory forces, particularly if individuals draw on the "environmental apparatus", namely their social milieu, above all the members of their family, whose support enables them to maintain a kind of equilibrium for a time before real suffering sets in.[12]

For Pearse and Crocker this was the point of departure for a much more far-reaching hypothesis: the researchers at the centre had found evidence that the environment functions in ways that go beyond the compensatory. When individuals make use of their environment in a state of health they can glean unimagined intensifying effects from this process of synthesis. And, our authors explain, they reserve the term "positive Health" for these very effects. Conversely, it had become evident that even the few healthy members – in purely physiological terms – were not always "functionally efficient" in the sense of being capable of effective action in unforeseen social situations. Here our authors make a striking leap: to them, this indicates that there are no born leaders; even leadership skills are the product of the "physical and social environment". Pearse and Crocker leave open what precisely terms such as "functional" and "efficient" mean for them. They merely suggest that we might conceive of positive health as a blend of psychological and physical resilience, a willingness to cooperate and learn, activity and flexibility. Remarkably, health also includes an ability to elicit the best in *others* on a situational basis. Ultimately, however, this use of the term conveys little more than a hazy notion of human potential: "We claim [...] that integration of the family developing in mutual synthesis with its environment will prove to be the biologically economic way of developing human potentiality – the way of health."[13]

The ideal life

In stylistic terms the rest of the book is less "scientific" than the first few chapters. It is also far more normative, foregrounding an at times almost mawkish narrative that seeks to demonstrate how human potential unfolds "biologically", that is, within the framework of the family and in the absence of artificial obstacles formed by social conventions and societal institutions. Pearse and Crocker accompany a young couple, Fred and Flo, during their first moments at the centre, which they find striking in its informality. Nothing, we are given to believe, is planned. Everything is self-administered, because, ultimately, the authors are out to find "evidence for spontaneous action in new circumstances". And such evidence is present in abundance: "In the Centre, the visitor is generally very surprised that what he sees before him is spontaneous action and not the result of program, persuasion or regulation. It is the conjunction of order with spontaneity that fazes him." Accordingly, the two new arrivals are not urged to become members but are instead "gently lapped" by the social activities at the centre.[14]

A few months later we meet the couple again; Flo is pregnant. The biologists monitor the pregnancy from a medical perspective, giving advice as required, though Flo also learns a great deal from other members. Another brief jump forward in time and the child has come into the world, moving up into the next "zone of mutuality", in other words migrating from the uterus to the familial "nest". The "weaning" process now starts, the gradual intensification of the child's interaction with the environment. This begins with "familiarised" meals as a supplement to his mother's milk,[15] while the ground is simultaneously laid for the family's gradual return to the centre – the "home" continues to expand. The child begins to walk, climb, and swim. At different times, in line with his individual propensities, he engages in various forms of physical coordination. He soon graduates from organic to social growth, continuously increasing his contact with others at the centre.

Although far removed from medical research, the next passages are perhaps the most important in the book. They begin with a lament on the school as institution. The latter, we are told, pays no heed to the child's individual "appetitive" phases, a failure that may even result in "allergic manifestations". The observations made at the centre, meanwhile, reveal that children bring tremendous focus to new activities if they themselves are allowed to determine their nature and duration.[16] Here one of the rare footnotes refers to a diagram in the appendix detailing the activities of an 11-year-old boy, which repays close scrutiny (Figure 4.2). It shows how, after an unsettled phase in which he tries out all the leisure activities at the centre in seemingly random fashion, the boy finds his way to his natural interests. These he then patiently develops. Along the diagram's temporal axis the contingency of his initial responses to the stimuli provided by the centre is gradually superseded by an individual pattern. Tellingly, this diagram is the only attempt ever published to formalize the centre's vitalizing effect. It is also the only figures-based representation of a "pattern of activity", as Pearse and Crocker call users' individual behaviours and learning curves.

This is particularly interesting because, from our authors' perspective, the individual learning process illustrated in the table is also making the child "altruistic". That is, children who undergo such processes in a self-determined way, yet in a group situation, develop a holistic perspective that is vital to learning consideration for others. This is why the centre's directors have mostly provided toys that facilitate "'competition' between the child and himself", such as trampolines. So the Peckham Experiment, the authors contend, by no means encouraged selfishness. Quite the opposite: it had turned all those involved into "demonstrators and instructors" for one another. In line with this, youths at the centre had demonstrated excellent social skills, as frequently noted by astonished visitors.[17]

Pearse and Crocker ultimately substantiate these claims with the help of just one highly suggestive motif. They go on to provide us with an account from the perspective of a child, one swinging from rope to rope with other children in the gymnasium, at close quarters, while adjusting his own route situationally to that of his fellows (Figure 4.3). This is quite different, the authors tell us, from a scenario in which just one child practises gymnastics

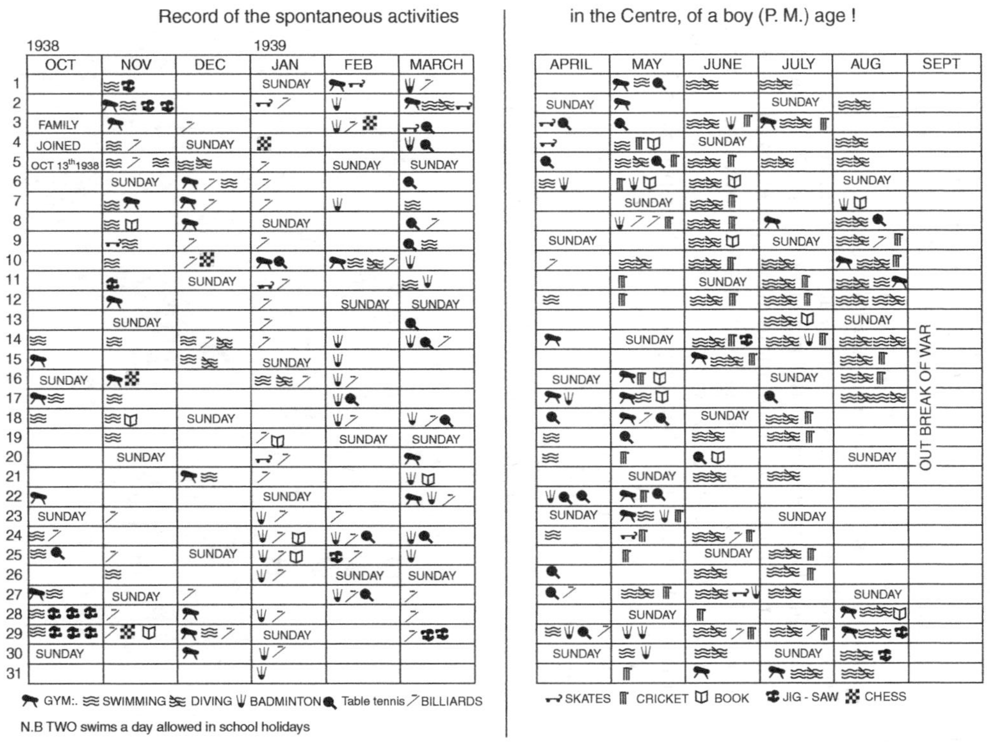

Record of the spontaneous activities

in the Centre, of a boy (P. M.) age !

Figure 4.2 Activities of an 11-year-old boy at the centre, October 1938 to August 1939. The pictograms show his development, month by month, into a swimmer and diver. This is interrupted by the outbreak of war. (Redrawn from: Innes H. Pearse and Lucy H. Crocker, *The Peckham Experiment. A Study of the Living Structure of Society.* London: Allen & Unwin, 1943, 318–319)

while being observed by the rest of the group, lined up along a bench. The swinging child is part of a "total situation", they write, "where mutual action is undertaken in awareness of a complex situation, that situation forever changing". This results in an "order arising out of the capacity of unintimidated human beings facultised to respond to the total situation". Pearse and Crocker implicitly extrapolated from this observation to the ideal society.[18]

Meanwhile, in their narrative, the youth's orbit grows beyond the bounds of the nuclear family "with its outer layer of casual contacts and acquaintances".[19] Here the text becomes rather prudish. It describes the youths' nightly bathing scenes, clearly a cipher for eroticism, which mark the genesis of the next couple-as-organism. Flirting too must be understood as mutual familiarization. This rapidly elicits a desire for a shared "hearth", emanating from the "urge to biological completion of the human organism".[20] The cycle is complete: the pair marry. The new – now anonymous, generalized – couple quickly sets about reproducing while availing itself of the knowledge provided by its social environment. We are given a synopsis of the pregnancy narrative from inception onwards. The account then terminates: older people, who are biologically uninteresting, are almost entirely absent from the book.

The Peckham Experiment concludes by returning to first principles. The focus now, according to the title of the conclusion, is on "social poverty". By this point at the latest the reader surely expects a systematic examination of the socioeconomic factors involved in the dysfunctions identified in the book.

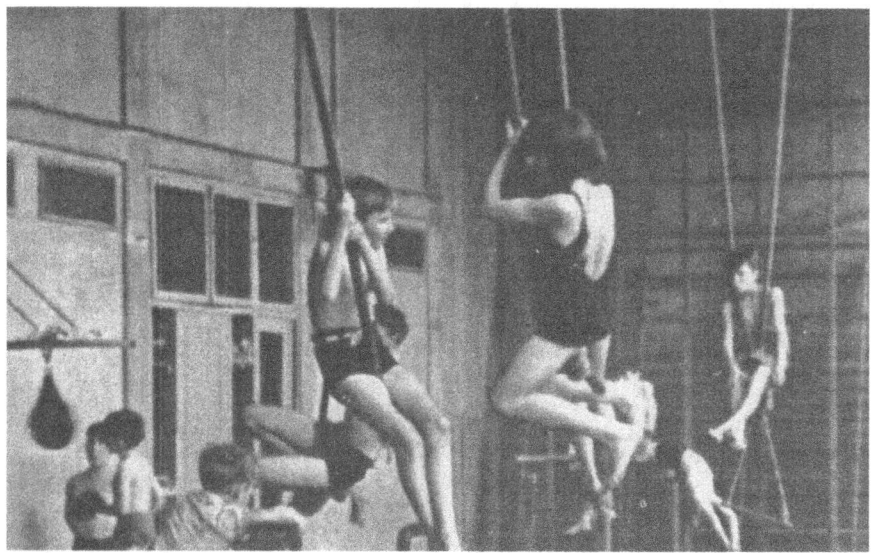

Figure 4.3 Children swinging on ropes in the centre's gymnasium – an example of an altruistic total situation, perhaps even of a living structure of society?
(Innes H. Pearse and Lucy H. Crocker, *The Peckham Experiment. A Study of the* Living *Structure of Society.* London: Allen & Unwin, 1943, 61, image detail)

Instead we are provided with a number of anonymous case histories. We learn, for example, about the monotonous daily routine of Mrs and Mr X – lonely, sick, socially inept individuals who do nothing but eat and sleep and whose existence rapidly improves when they begin to attend the centre. Mrs X, for example, becomes active, sewing her own clothes while her children develop pleasant personalities. This final section in particular – at least at first sight – foregrounds users' self-empowerment. The centre has enhanced their "ability to formulate [their] needs or to go out in search of them".[21] But this had never been an end in itself: "All the chances offered by the Centre [...] are there to be woven by the family itself into the contextual fabric of its gathering experience." The conclusion, then, characterizes the PHC as the "nucleus of a Society the structure of which is neither 'planned' nor 're-constructed' but living; that is to say growing, developing, differentiating, as the result of the mutual synthesis of its component cells – its homes". Pearse and Crocker conclude apodictically: "The individual is but an evolutionary dead-end – a cul-de-sac of biological energy seeking canalisation."[22]

Culture and cultivation

Like its predecessor, *A Case for Action, The Peckham Experiment* too presents us with a fusion of ideas that do not appear to belong together. Based on evolutionary biology, at times even on "cosmic" suppositions, the book argues that the priority of any project of social reform must be to dismantle impediments to the flow of information between human beings. Within modern civilization, the authors assert, these hamper the realization of species-specific potentials. This enthusiasm for spontaneous, unregulated ordering processes is quite out of sync with the euphoric embrace of planning that researchers often regard as the cross-national hallmark of the early 1940s. Yet it would be wrong to conclude that the project had prompted Pearse and Crocker to embrace a form of subject-centred empowerment *avant la lettre*. We need only recall the anti-individualism so characteristic of their thinking or their strong tendency to naturalize the (nuclear) family and community.

In any case, the book shows that the centre was not the scene of the rigorously scientific social experiment some commentators continue to perceive. First, the project was replete with confirmation bias, "data" being processed in such a way as to pre-empt the findings. The best examples here are the membership criteria, family examinations and family consultations. The latter two in particular helped create the very entities whose spontaneous growth the Peckham researchers sought to record. Second, there was no yardstick by which to gauge the centre's effects. There was no control group; in their book a least, Pearse and Crocker never concerned themselves with those local residents who did not wish to become members or, being single, were unable to. And they failed to ask themselves to what degree the self-selection of their social sample diminished the representativeness of their observations. They said nothing about the fact that the centre must surely have attracted people who were open to new experiences and thus more inclined to embrace the knowledge on offer. Third, we might dispute the significance of a study, for just over four years, of a heavily fluctuating social group. Above all, though, in light of the short data collection period, we might question how the authors came up with the idealized reproductive cycle that structures their book. In fact they had a general tendency to leave their readers in the dark about the development of their ideas.

So the question arises as to why the researchers could not see that, through their experiment, they were to some extent producing the "natural" phenomena they wished to observe. This is all the more striking in that their search for the living structure of society made political and economic issues seem secondary, as evident in the proverbial nutshell in Pearse and Crocker's rope-swinging scenario, cited by a number of authors since the 1940s to exemplify the lessons learned from the centre.[23] Through this scenario the authors sought to convey a nature that continuously allocates every human being a place in accordance with his abilities, taking no account of the fact that the exercising children manage to avoid colliding only on the condition of sufficient room for all (we might also say resources or money). Thus, anyone endowing the gymnasium scenario with significance to society as a whole risked losing sight of the relative poverty afflicting the people of South London, if not the Peckham residents themselves. In fact, *The Peckham Experiment* mentioned only in passing and without presenting any supporting evidence that higher wages could do little to alleviate most people's plight.[24] But to anticipate a point I will develop in more detail later on, many Peckham residents went to the centre because, even to individuals well above the poverty line, basic medical care was often very costly, if not virtually unaffordable elsewhere.[25] From the Peckham scholars' point of view, however, they lived in a state of dormant biological potential rather than economic constraint.

I have no wish to deny that the centre was a genuine source of enrichment for many of its users.[26] But a reading of *The Peckham Experiment*, and this makes the book so interesting from an historical point of view, reveals that the researchers' perception of the social processes unfolding within the centre entailed certain preconceived ideas about the laws governing these processes. We need only think of their certainty that the *biological* nuclear family was the only relevant social entity. At no point did they discuss the possible influence that other forms of close coexistence – the extended family, workplace friendships, solidarity-based political communities – might have had on centre users' conduct.[27] In general terms it appears as though Pearse and Crocker (and no doubt Scott Williamson as well) had immunized themselves against the problem that users' lives outside the centre – with all their constraints and specificities – simply continued in the absence of interference, in other words, that their laboratory was from the outset culturally "contaminated".

This reinforces the need to explain why the Peckham researchers sought to help nature along with methods that – if one wishes to establish this problematic boundary in the first place – one would allocate to the realm of culture. The experiment continually created *meaning* (the family consultation being a prime example) with the goal of prompting users to engage in activities deemed natural. Pearse and Crocker, however, did not see it this way. In their eyes, a conversation between doctors and users, which – however friendly it may have been – involved a highly unequal distribution of symbolic capital, was a form of quasi-physiological input. This made their own medical advice seem less like a form of instruction than a contribution to "mutual synthesis", as especially apparent in light of Pearse's and Crocker's aforementioned forays into a semantic field revolving around nurture. The researchers believed themselves to be playing the role of "cultivators" at the centre, providing the right soil for young plants. This could mean anything from testing blood values to providing tips on nutrition: "To gain health one must till the soil, sow, wait and watch before reaping the harvest of health we set out to cultivate."[28] But the agrarian symbolism, the tilling of fallow potential, cannot disguise the paternalistic sense of superiority inherent in these metaphors: those who cultivate others, even in a biological sense, must inevitably be more cultivated themselves.

Before examining the provenance of the biologistic mindset revealed in these quotations, I would like to turn briefly to the form of expression chosen by the authors of *The Peckham Experiment*. The success of their book outside the scientific community is no doubt due in part to the highly readable but hazy narrative of familiarization within the centre.[29] Pearse and Crocker deployed multiple techniques to undergird the validity of their statements, even linking together several types of media: in their book tables lend support to allegorical narratives, which are in turn verified by photographs. In addition, narrative style and perspective often shift. On many occasions the boundary between matter-of-fact research report and fiction becomes blurred. The intake interview, for example, is presented through the directors' direct speech; elsewhere the reader listens to users' thoughts; often, the boldest of assertions are placed in the mouths of visitors. Particularly striking are the many passages that suddenly use the present tense, as if to emphasize the spontaneity of members' actions. Pearse and Crocker, moreover, had a predilection for case histories, which they presented – without further elaboration – as *pars pro toto* of members' interwoven patterns of activity. These techniques were more than just tools of popularization. In fact they appear to have been attempts to convey the holistic view of the centre that our authors had embraced by this stage. For it is hard to miss the fact – and even the figures in the appendix do nothing to change this – that Pearse and Crocker were sceptical of presentational techniques focused on formalization, particularly those substantiated by statistics, which they viewed as mechanistic.

Interwar holisms

Both these tendencies, the attempt to cultivate human beings in a biological sense and the rejection of a purely quantifying scientific practice, are more than chance phenomena. This is evident if – in contrast to the existing literature on Peckham – we take account of Scott Williamson's and Pearse's research on Graves' disease, goitre and thyroid hormones, in which they were engaged in parallel with their work at the first centre on Queen's Road and in the early 1930s. The two doctors were certainly performing basic histological research through, for example, microscopic studies of cell structure in the thyroid.[30] Their work on the thyroid in particular, however, also provided the conceptual prerequisite for their odd leaps between physiological theories of development and the interpretation of the social realm as growth medium.

At least since the publication of Robert McCarrisson's research on vitamin deficiency in the early 1920s, scientists had been aware of the importance of the thyroid to embryonic growth and metabolic processes generally. Around the same time, in a much-noticed experiment, Julian Huxley, later an influential patron of the Peckham centre,[31] had shown that administering thyroid hormones could trigger the metamorphosis of the axolotl – a Mexican caudate that remains permanently in the larval stage – into a full-grown salamander. The hormone thyroxin seemed to exercise a decisive influence on the development of organisms – at least in the opinion of the *Daily Mail*, which speculated that Huxley had discovered the elixir of life.[32] Furthermore, during this period progress in endocrinology and the widespread interest in hormones and their function as messenger substances engendered a conception of the organism that to some extent anticipated modern information theory, a conception akin to the PHC researchers' ideas in certain respects, in that it construed the body as a homeostatic system of interdependent organ functions (the term homeostasis being first used by Walter B. Cannon in 1932). A system that responds flexibly to external stimuli, the body seemed capable of continually regulating and stabilizing its own "internal milieu".[33]

But research on the thyroid also bolstered the political resonance of nutritional science. It initiated the investigation of deficiency diseases such as rickets, a key topic in the debate on military recruits mentioned earlier.[34] Overall, in fact, the findings of nutritional physiology heavily influenced debates on welfare in the interwar period, one example being the nutritional advice provided by the British Medical Association (BMA), whose guidelines infiltrated the human needs indices of poverty statistics.[35] Rowntree's famous poverty line also had a dietary dimension: he defined poverty as falling short of the minimum physiological conditions under which "physical efficiency" could be maintained.

So it was in keeping with the times that Scott Williamson and Pearse linked their research at the centre – albeit in an increasingly metaphorical way – with the social components of preventive medicine, specifically, with the notion of enriching the individual's familial milieu with free-floating knowledge, and with the idea that the "digestion" of this knowledge fostered human beings' development. Like McCarrisson, with whom they corresponded repeatedly in the early 1930s,[36] they also tested out these ideas through animal experiments.

Scott Williamson believed he had observed a lower incidence of illness in rat "families" than in individual animals grouped together randomly,[37] and the centre must have appeared to him as the application of this experiment to human beings.

It was, in other words, recent medical findings that prompted Pearse and Scott Williamson to study everyday social life, human relationships and communication within the centre, in which they had begun to work in the 1920s, viewing members' interaction and development through the epistemological lens of immunology and, to an even greater extent, nutritional physiology. They were in fact never to deviate from this perspective. This heightened their awareness of interdependencies and interactions rather than essences and awakened their interest in environmental factors.

It is, however, difficult to exactly estimate how much of this style of thought was the product of their reading and how much they came up with themselves. Scott Williamson, Pearse and Crocker, as mentioned already, used virtually no footnotes in their books and provided their readers with sparse bibliographical information. The classical approach to reconstructing the history of ideas, then, is closed to us.[38] Generally speaking, the Peckham directors' interests overlapped with broader discourses of holism in the early 1930s, which were often underpinned by anti-mechanistic assumptions in much the same way as their own ideas. Medical holism, which was widespread in Britain, for example, may be interpreted as a critique of methods, as a call for a more integrated form of medical practice. Many older generalists feared that the specialization of laboratory medicine would irreparably fragment the sciences while also abolishing certain privileges enjoyed by the medical profession.[39] But even beyond the life sciences this was a time when supposedly simplifying and materialist approaches came under fire and perspectives rooted in theories of social interdependence found approval, though these frequently blurred into esotericism.[40] We can make a connection between the Peckham researchers' interest in the relationships between human beings and an anthropocentric turn that crosscut countries and disciplines. Between the world wars calls came from various quarters for the humanization of industrial society, for an ecological focus on the whole person in light of his emotional embeddedness in his social milieu[41] – whether in the young discipline of industrial sociology or the Chicago School's research on urban life and migration. This sometimes culminated in a kind of progressive cultural criticism, as in the case of American planning theorist Lewis Mumford, who was to play a minor part in the centre's post-war history, and whose widely read publications justified the imperative for planning with reference to an organic ideal of community.[42] Of course, there are major differences between the proposed interventions derived from such critiques. These ranged from the rigid behaviourist control of the population in the authoritarian states of the time to more or less Hippocratic efforts intended to lay the ground for the social organism's natural growth, an approach better able to attract support in Britain in the 1930s.

Eugenics, evolution and community

Even the evolutionary biology in *The Peckham Experiment* was less eccentric at the time than we might initially imagine, overlapping with the ideas of those British researchers who, like Huxley, were closely associated with the Eugenics Society. In the years immediately following the closure of the centre on St Mary's Road this institution found itself facing strong pressure to change. Not only had the society chalked up virtually no political successes more than 25 years after its foundation, but it seemed more unlikely than ever to do so: within the British public sphere eugenics was interpreted as the cience of heredity, if not selection through sterilization (of the kind rejected, of course, by Scott Williamson and Pearse). As such, particularly from the perspective of left-wing commentators, eugenics appeared to be an obstacle to political reforms.[43] During the period of planning for the second centre, Eugenics Society representatives sought to stake out their differences from so-called mainline eugenics, making their understanding of the relationship between nature and nurture markedly more nuanced and engendering a reform eugenics sensitized to social issues. This rapidly became established on the institutional level, in part because it had a good deal in common with the planning movement of the second half of the 1930s (more on this later).[44] In 1930, for example, William Beveridge, director of the London School of Economics and Political Science (LSE) and later pioneer of the welfare state, made Lancelot Hogben head of a new department of social biology, which investigated the relationship between biological and social factors in shaping society and explored the policy implications. In much the same way as Pearse and Scott Williamson, Hogben believed social hurdles could impede the realization of individual genetic potential, with researchers in the field making copious use of animal experiments to prove it.

Though they barely mentioned other researchers, the directors of the Peckham Experiment are likely to have viewed their own findings against the background of these attempts to reduce biological "wastage". This is especially probable given that influential researchers such as Huxley and Lord Thomas Horder, president of the Eugenics Society between 1935 and 1949, personally endorsed the PHC's work. But some of the fault lines of the 1940s are already in evidence despite the fact that Horder, a traditional doctor, believed the centre was mirroring his own efforts to maintain the personal link between doctor and patient. For reform eugenics also contributed to the growing importance of specialized proto-sociological studies on the basis of statistical methods. For example, in 1933–1934, in a large-scale study, Hogben's department at the LSE had investigated the influence of the school system on the development of pupils in London. This marked a trend that, shortly after the publication of *The Peckham Experiment*, inspired methodological reservations about the PHC directors' approach, a development that was to prove fatal to the centre over the medium term, as we shall see.

But initially it was the common ground that predominated, and this included the understanding of social integration and evolution that pervades Pearse and Crocker's book. Many members of the "visible college" of the 1930s, who were bound together by their sociobiological interests,[45] such as neurologist C.S. Sherrington and, once again, Julian Huxley, assumed that higher organisms were distinguished by a pronounced individuality on the one hand and their outstanding capacity for stabilization and integration on the other.[46] At the same time they began to perceive the process of evolution less and less as a struggle for survival and increasingly as a series of cooperative acts. For many British biologists it was thus quite possible to use models derived from the observation of nature to understand social organization. In fact, they sometimes failed to make it clear when they were referring to mere analogies. Huxley in particular tended – for a time – to infer a natural telos of human social forms from the so-called "eusocial" behaviour of state-forming species. The human being seemed to stand at the pinnacle of nature given his capacity to deploy his own highly developed personality altruistically to the benefit of his community.

This idea had the additional advantage of making the discipline of biology highly attractive to the interwar British elite. Those in favour of maintaining the status quo could use such an interpretation of evolution to back up their arguments, contending that "cultivated" individuals were better suited to leadership positions within mass society. In any case, the latest findings of the natural sciences could legitimize the building of bridges between older Victorian educational ideals, which sought to improve individual morality and character, and the optimistic scientism of the 1920s and 1930s. The "scientific humanism" advocated by Huxley and others within the political sphere on the basis of these theories fortified a bourgeois elite in their meritocratic value system while simultaneously lending it a scientific aura. Much like Pearse and Scott Williamson, many evolutionary biologists believed their intellectual work was expediting the integration of a community.[47] Scientists embodied quasi-natural progress: they lived exemplary lives that seemed to demonstrate the compatibility of clashing norms central to British social ethics – such as "integration" and "individualism".

Importantly, this did not stop a number of experimental biologists from interpreting the process of evolution through the lens of democracy. Hogben and geneticist John B.S. Haldane in particular believed that the unfolding of human genetic and cultural variability formed the basis for a well-integrated society of fulfilled individuals. (In contrast to Pearse and Scott Williamson, however, both emphasized that this required fair starting conditions that must be achieved through political action.) Their reform socialism, underpinned by evolutionary ideas, thus assumed that human diversity was of benefit to democracy as long as it remained subject to mediation. Conversely, collectivist societies that strove to achieve complete homogeneity, but also those with a tendency towards excessive specialization, seemed to lose their capacity for cooperation and their flexibility – and this was associated with an evolutionary dead end.[48]

Scott Williamson's, Pearse's and Crocker's concepts of life, nurture, development and cultivation, then, were reflective of widespread debates of their time. And it was these same concepts that also laid the ground for the specific way in which they dealt with centre users, a topic to which we now turn.[49] After 1935, the centre directors increasingly focused their attention on social interactions. In doing so, they were encountering essentially unforeseen phenomena, turning the "anti-specialism" they shared with the holists and scientific humanists of the day into outright hostility to science understood as the mere registering of facts. But first, this anti-specialism motivated Scott Williamson's attempts to transmit a simplified version of his own findings to the participants in his experiment. In the mid 1930s he began to deliver a kind of public soliloquy at the centre on the scientist as a human type, as we will see in a moment. Scott Williamson was clearly trying to walk a fine line between the (isolating) life of the expert and (individuality-threatening) over-integration. This seemed to be the only way to avoid hampering the progressive differentiation of the centre community and thus the qualitative "growth" of humanity as a whole.

Notes

1 Crocker's main contribution was to write the chapters dealing with children and young people. Both also worked up draft texts by Scott Williamson: Pearse to Winfrey, August 8, 1942, WL, SA/PHC/B.4/5/1.
2 Pearse and Crocker, *The Peckham Experiment*, 5.
3 Ibid., 10.
4 Documents created during the preparation of these tables show that initially the plan was to contrast the state of health of housewives and women in employment but (apparently for want of significant differences) this idea was dropped for the final publication: Tabulations of patients, c. 1937–1939, WL, SA/PHC/B.3/5/2.
5 Pearse and Crocker, *The Peckham Experiment*, 307–310.
6 Ibid., quotations: 16–18, 21, 24.
7 Ibid., 25–26.
8 Ibid., 37.
9 Ibid., 42.
10 Ibid., 205, 81, 71, 67–70, 75.
11 Ibid., 85, 81.
12 Ibid., 205, 81, 71, 67–70, 75, 103–104. With the help of a case history Pearse and Crocker illustrate how effectively the family examination can diagnose such disorders: it was not until they put their heads together that the members of one particular family discovered the causes of their diabetes, and this helped diminish the conflicts between them: "a solvent for both bio-chemical and social disorder in this family". Ibid., 109.
13 Ibid., 113, 119, 120, 122.
14 Ibid., 125, 128, 134.
15 Ibid., 150–152, 164. "Familiarised" because, unlike industrially produced baby food, the mother herself has consumed them during her pregnancy.
16 Ibid., 188, 201.
17 Ibid., 181, 195, 204, 206.
18 This, at least, is one reading of a footnote in which they make a connection with England's disastrous road accident statistics: traffic is overregulated, preventing

individuals from developing an awareness of its totality. Ibid., 193, 192. The rope-swinging scenario also appears in the photographic chapter (Figure 4.3).

19 Ibid., 207.
20 Ibid., 255. Pearse and Crocker argue that it is particularly important not to limit contact between youths in accordance with gender or age, as common in many youth organizations, as this diminishes the potential for biologically complementary partners to encounter one another. Geneticists, the authors assert, are overly focused on breeding, but in fact what really matters is to enable nature to unfold without restriction – and this includes facilitating love across social strata (ibid., 228 f.). Biology, then, takes priority over social conventions, and this also applies to institutionalized partnerships: Pearse and Crocker tend to refer to marriage in a figurative sense. On the other hand they favour monogamy and approve of (female) virginity prior to a long-term partnership – for "biological" reasons. They also reject prostitution and masturbation. The latter, they surmise, may be the result of worm infestation: ibid., 211.
21 Ibid., 250–253, 289
22 Ibid., 290, 298.
23 See for example Alison Stallibrass, *The Self-Respecting Child* (London: Thames and Hudson), 22; Colin Ward, "'A Laboratory of Anarchy'. A Comparative Anthology", *Anarchy* 6 (1966): 59; and Leila Berg, "Moving Towards Self Government", in *Children's Rights. Towards the Liberation of the Child*, ed. Julian Hall, (London: Panther, 1972), 27.
24 Pearse and Crocker, *The Peckham Experiment*, 274.
25 According to the synopsis of an interview with Pam Elven, British Library, Millennium Memory Bank, 1999, C900/05095A C1.
26 See Chapter 8.
27 There were evidently no political events of any kind at the centre; but none of the PHC publications elucidate whether and if so how these were prohibited.
28 First eight months. May–Dec. 1935, WL, SA/PHC/B.3/8/1, 10.
29 Pearse and Crocker, *The Peckham Experiment*, 246.
30 George Scott Williamson and Innes H. Pearse, "Evidence drawn from a study of the therapeutics of Graves' Disease, of two functions in the thyroid physiology", *Quarterly Journal of Medicine* 22 (1928): 21–31. I note in passing that at this time Scott Williamson was also working on the Wassermann reaction, that is, the serology of syphilis, with the help of which Ludwik Fleck developed his theory of the genesis of scientific facts, a significant source of stimulation for the present work.
31 Huxley repeatedly praised the PHC: Julian Huxley, *Scientific Research and Social Needs* (London: Watts & Co., 1934), 101–103; "The National Physique", *The Times*, November 13, 1936; "Manalive. A New Biological Study. The Pioneer Health Centre", *The Times*, June 4, 1939. Conversely, his role as a pioneering figure for the Peckham actors is evident in the poem composed by Peckham poet and eccentric William Margrie in the mid 1930s: "Arise proud Peckham, and lead the world / Tell all the nations that art's not dead / Peckham has arisen and all is well / Peckham's health shrine stands firm on St Mary's Hill. / Nuffield's name, the brains of Pearse and Scott, / *Huxley's science* and Lady Stanley's smile / Have combined to make Peckham what she is, / The pioneer of Freedom, health and laughter. / Not marble, nor the gilded monuments / Of princes shall outlive this powerful shrine. / Peckham wrestles with Rome for mankind's soul. / Peckham points the way to Superman. / Not Mussolini's scowl or Hitler's frown, / But Peckham's smile shall win the immortal Crown" (TNA, MH 52/159, my emphasis).
32 Julian Huxley, *Memories* (Harmondsworth: Penguin Books, 1972), 125–126.

33 Mark Jackson, *The Age of Stress. Science and the Search for Stability* (Oxford: Oxford University Press, 2013), 70–75; Jakob Tanner, "'Weisheit des Körpers' und soziale Homöostase. Physiologie und das Konzept der Selbstregulation", in *Physiologie und industrielle Gesellschaft. Studien zur Verwissenschaftlichung des Körpers im 19. und 20. Jahrhundert*, ed. Jakob Tanner and Philipp Sarasin (Frankfurt: Suhrkamp, 1998), 129–169.

34 The cause of rickets, a lack of vitamin D, had been discovered by Edward Mellanby in 1919. Much like Huxley, he was to play an important role for the PHC in the 1940s.

35 Gazeley, *Poverty in Britain*, 89–90.

36 See the correspondence in the WL, SA/PHC/F.16/4.

37 Pearse, *The Quality of Life*, 162.

38 There are, however, indications that – in addition to the thinkers mentioned above – they were heavily influenced by South African evolutionary theorist and politician Jan Smuts. Scott Williamson later tried without success to get Smuts to write a foreword to *The Peckham Experiment* (see: To General Smuts, "Author of Holism" [early 1940s], WL, SA/PHC/D.1/7/8). In his 1926 magnum opus *Holism and Evolution* Smuts had tried to demonstrate that both the natural and social worlds tended towards the formation of ever more complex "wholes". He also regarded the British empire as a whole and argued that only white people had reached a developmental stage facilitative of the empire's development. In 1935 this prompted botanist Arthur Tansley (who coined the term "ecosystem") to assail him for misusing "vegetational" concepts: Peder Anker, *Imperial Ecology. Environmental Order in the British Empire* (Cambridge, MA: Harvard University Press, 2001), 118–156.

39 Christopher Lawrence, "Still Incommunicable: Clinical Holists and Medical Knowledge in Interwar Britain", in Lawrence and George Weisz, eds., *Greater than the Parts*, 94–111; and Dorothy Porter, "Social Medicine and the New Society: Medicine and Scientific Humanism in mid-Twentieth Century Britain", *Journal of Historical Sociology* 9 (1996): 168–187.

40 An example here is Kurt Goldstein, whose studies of soldiers with brain injuries had sensitized him to the organism's compensatory potential, prompting him to define health as the ability to realize one's own nature – strikingly similar to Scott Williamson's definitional efforts. His 1934 book *The Organism* dealt with the response to natural stability, linking its optimization with self-realization, which he regarded as the precondition for harmonious interaction with the cosmos: Anne Harrington, *Reenchanted Science. Holism in German Culture. From Wilhelm II to Hitler* (Princeton, NJ: Princeton University Press, 1996); and Mitchell G. Ash, *Gestalt Psychology in German Culture 1890–1967. Holism and the Quest for Objectivity* (Cambridge: Cambridge University Press, 1995).

41 Timo Luks, "The Factory as Environment. Social Engineering and the Ecology of Industrial Workplaces in Inter-War Germany", *European Review of History: Revue europeenne d'histoire* 20 (2013): 271–285.

42 Casey Nelson Blake, *Beloved Community. The Cultural Criticism of Randolph Bourne, Van Wyck Brooks, & Lewis Mumford* (Chapel Hill/London: University of North Carolina Press, 1990).

43 Pauline M. Mazumdar, *Eugenics, Human Genetics, and Human Failings: The Eugenics Society, its Sources and its Critics in Britain* (London: Routledge, 1992); and Greta Jones, "Eugenics and Social Policy between the Wars", *Historical Journal* 25 (1982): 717–728. Specifically on the eugenicists' "International", whose comparative perspective reinforced British critics' unease, see: Stefan Kühl, *For the Betterment of the Race. The Rise and Fall of the International Movement for Eugenics and Racial Hygiene* (New York: Palgrave Macmillan, 2013); and Marius Turda, *Modernism and Eugenics* (Basingstoke: Palgrave Macmillan, 2010).

44 Chris Renwick, "Eugenics, Population Research, and Social Mobility Studies in Early and Mid-Twentieth-Century Britain", *The Historical Journal* 59 (2016): 845–867.

45 Gary Werskey, *The Visible College. A Collective Biography of British Scientists and Socialists of the 1930s* (London: Free Association, 1988).

46 Roger Smith, "Biology and Values in Interwar Britain: C. S. Sherrington, Julian Huxley and the Vision of Progress", *Past & Present* 178 (2003): 226.

47 One of the ways they did this was by popularizing their knowledge – Hogben spoke of "self-education" – by means of readable monographs; the young Penguin Books publishing house was of considerable significance here.

48 Marianne Sommer, "Die Biologie der Demokratie im Wissenschaftlichen Humanismus", in *Wissenschaft und Demokratie*, ed. Michael Hagner (Frankfurt: Suhrkamp, 2012), 51–68.

49 Here we should note another ideology that helped form the backdrop to many British reform projects, even if there is no direct connection with the PHC. Pearse and Crocker shared with the Quakers – who counted among their number many influential social reformers – the idea of a conflict-free community of individuals, whose potential only emerges through social cooperation. The harmonious cosmos of the natural world evoked by the PHC researchers is strikingly reminiscent of the Quakers' idea of creation, while their notion of biological potential recalls the "inner light" that many Quakers believe every individual should be able to express freely. Still instructive in this regard is: John Child, "Quaker Employers and Industrial Relations", *Sociological Review* 12 (1964): 293–315.

5 Looking through the bioscope

Research and social interaction in the pre-war centre (1935–1939)

In the spring of 1935, on St Mary's Road, evolutionary thinking sensitized to processes of cooperation came up against the reality of the district of Peckham. By the following year, in the official annual report, for the first time Scott Williamson enthusiastically described the unique opportunity to observe life in the Pioneer Health Centre. In particular he highlighted how close one could get to one's objects of study:

> It is only necessary for them [the doctors] to come down one flight of stairs, and they are able to observe or take part in the general life of the Centre. [...] Perhaps never before has there been for any doctor or any scientist a field so rich and so varied in which to work, nor a group of such willing subjects, eager to co-operate. The problem which continually faces the research worker here is not "what line will be most likely to give results" – but rather – "how to cope with such wealth of new material".[1]

The most remarkable phrase in this quotation is "to cope". It implies that the Peckham researchers were overwhelmed by the "material" surrounding them the moment they left their laboratories. They had suffered something of a reality shock. In order to further determine why they increasingly focused on the spontaneous social interactions of the centre members, it is crucial to follow up this particular lead.

Hence, in what follows I seek to reconstruct events at the centre during the first few weeks and months after it was opened. On a number of occasions this will involve correlating statements made by different individuals from different time periods, such as letters from this initial phase and memoirs from the 1980s. While this rules out a neat narrative, in contrast to the Peckham researchers' official publications it reveals that their findings on social self-organization, for which the experiment is known today, were the result of a sometimes painful learning process triggered by their encounter with the centre members.

Data collection

Reconstructing the medical work done at the centre presents no great difficulties. It was fairly conventional. The few surviving family records detailing the findings of the initial and follow-up examinations are unavailable due to data protection laws. But a number of blank datasheets and pre-printed forms for patients' medical history from the 1930s have survived.[2] These noted the adults' place of birth, name, address and occupation, and recorded data on all family members' height, muscle tone, teeth, eyes, hearing, skin, glands and bone structure. The only unusual elements are columns for "mentality", "education", and "language".[3] These demonstrate that the doctors were making psychosocial observations.

We can also reconstruct the routines of the medical personnel, at least for the *post-war* period, with the help of a manual from 1948. This shows that when it came to creating ideal starting conditions for social syntheses – at least with respect to the work of *some* centre employees – the directors considered a high degree of procedural standardization appropriate. They clearly thought these staff members capable of coping with relatively unspontaneous, quasi-bureaucratic processes without suffering a sense of alienation,[4] detailing a seamless chain of actions encompassing 35 tasks, including precise instructions on when to hand users an examination gown.[5] A task breakdown was also produced for staff at the reception desk. This specified, for example, how to make appointments for the family consultation and when to send out reminders about impending annual examinations.[6] There was even a uniform colour code for the types of ink used for the pre-printed forms. This distinguished between illnesses, developmental stages (in the case of children), prenatal consultations, hospital stays and so on. All of this related to the administration of the experiment or to its medical dimension in the narrower sense. However, almost 15 years after the start of an investigation into the structure of society the comment accompanying the purple ink was: "'sociological' – not yet in use."[7]

As far as the records of members work on their own potential is concerned, the evidence is generally unclear. To all appearances, here the main role was played by the so-called "curators", the members of staff responsible for the centre's social spaces and activities. Towards the end of the 1940s they too were provided with recommendations, though these were less detailed. Evidently, the curators and their assistants (often students) showed new members around and informed them about the building's facilities, the principle of self-service governing the cafeteria, but also their own role: they helped coordinate larger-scale activities and had to look after furniture and equipment, carrying out small repairs for example. One significant task was to facilitate contact: "[W]hile walking around, the opportunity should be taken to introduce a new member to any member they meet, where that is possible."[8]

Oddly enough nothing in the lists indicates that the curators helped with the research. For in retrospect this was portrayed as their main task, for example by Alison Stallibrass, assistant from 1936 to 1939 to Lucy Crocker, one of the centre's first curators. In the mid 1970s Stallibrass described how the curators moved ceaselessly through the building. This had ensured the continuous dispersal of the children within the centre, exposing them to an ever-changing variety of stimuli. As we have seen, most activities within the centre cost money; the grown-ups acquired the requisite tickets in the cafeteria, while children could get them free of charge, upon request, from the curator. These paper tokens served as receipts but also as a means of data collection, according to Stallibrass. For instance, a ticket was required to gain entry to the changing rooms on the ground floor, which in turn led to the pool and the gymnasium. Anyone taking toys or sports equipment from one of the storage boxes scattered throughout the building had to write their name (or in the case of small children their initials) on their ticket and put it in a special box.[9] The tickets, which could thus be matched with individuals and days, were collected every evening and filed away with the family records. Scott Williamson and Pearse liked to be photographed with the latter documents (Figure 5.1). Yet there is nothing in the sources to indicate any systematic, quantitative analysis of this material. The plan for a "centre key" – an individual copper coin for every member, which would have opened turnstiles and might have been used for more precise data collection – came to nothing.[10]

While the researchers seem to have been committed to recording the activities of specific individuals, we learn nothing about how they established the existence of the spontaneous social order described in *The Peckham Experiment*. The official publications never mention who exactly had made the socio-biological observations within the centre and how such complex processes as increasing social integration and mutual stimulation were registered. It would, for example, have been conceivable to produce statistical correlation analyses of the family members' activity patterns. Instead the researchers mostly backed up their case with anecdotes. Yet they failed to reveal how they noted these down, for example, what aids to memory they used.[11]

Perhaps unsurprisingly, then, the programmatic texts published during the centre's planning phase provide no indication that the researchers had given any thought to developing a consistent methodology to record natural, spontaneous, interpersonal syntheses at the centre. As we saw in *The Case for Action*, in 1931 no plans had yet been made to facilitate users' self-organization, let alone observe it scientifically. A staff list reveals that as late as 1934, just a few months before the inauguration of the centre, the directors had appointed an "organizer" for the women's section and one trainer each for the gymnasium and swimming pool. They also envisaged a division of users into lay and advanced courses.[12] To all appearances, at this point Scott Williamson and Pearse had yet to start viewing certain practices – courses, achievement tests, organization – as biological impediments. This changed rapidly in the first few months after the centre's opening.

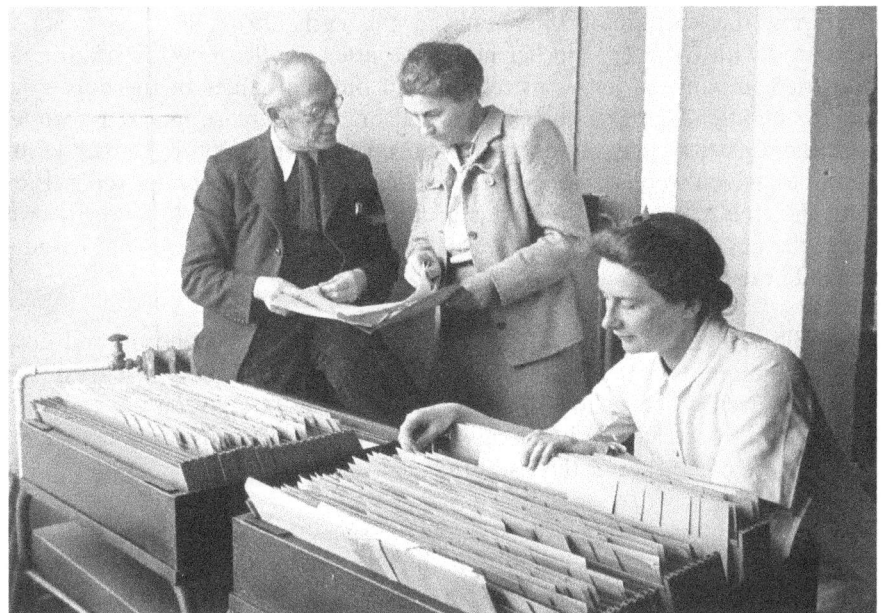

Figure 5.1 Scott Williamson and Pearse in the late 1940s with their material – discussing a "pattern of activity"?
(Axel Scott-Samuel, *Total Participation, Total Health: Reinventing the Peckham Health Centre for the 1990s*. Edinburgh: Scottish Academic Press, 1990, 18)

Chaos and order

As we have seen, the annual reports of 1935 and 1936 paint a harmonious picture of the activities at the new centre. There is nothing surprising about this: we are talking about status reports for nervous backers. Conversely, the participants' retrospective accounts – from a safe distance – mention substantial teething difficulties. *The Peckham Experiment* merely indicates that initially the adult members were passive and shy and that the children's boisterous behaviour in particular hindered the researchers' work. But we get an idea of the full extent of the problem in *The Quality of Life*, Pearse's last book from 1979. It dedicates a key chapter to the first few months, one headed "Chaos". Here Pearse describes things probably better kept from financial sponsors. Theft was a major problem initially. Cushions were torn and the glass walls were plastered with unauthorized items. The children used the heavy glass ashtrays for "curling"; the new-fangled sliding windows were eminently suited to playing "railways". In the meantime the apathetic parents nursed their beers in the cafeteria instead of, as hoped, taking advantage of the activities on offer. More than once, Pearse admits, in light of these realities she had felt the need "to say 'don't', and/or remove from sight and reach the instruments designed to be at the disposal of all the members". Particularly towards evening things had become intolerable: "Chaos raged for many months."[13]

During the writing of this book in the early 1970s Pearse repeatedly conferred with Crocker.[14] In her notes the latter recalled how, as curator, she had tried in vain for weeks merely to find out the names of the boisterous, larking children. Crocker installed herself on the staircase in order to intercept them as they played and sign them up for swimming and other leisure activities, which were supposed to take place regularly and under supervision, with the children subdivided by age group. None of the children ever showed up at the appointed time. For Crocker, this was the start of a "long period of absolute misery":

> [W]hat we did was to walk and walk and walk round and up and down the building – watching the destruction, powerless to stop it, harassed by every well wisher who came into the building. "Can't you do something to stop these children breaking everything up?" The answer of course was that we could, but at the risk of driving them out.[15]

It is important to note the sense of powerlessness expressed in this quotation. Crocker became painfully aware that she was dependent on the centre users' collaboration, in other words, that she could not punish them or force them to become active. It also dawned on her that the last thing the children wanted after school was further regulation, particularly of their urge to move. It therefore proved necessary, Crocker noted, to grant the children access to activities on a case-by-case basis.[16] Initially, however, this appears to have been a straightforward safety issue rather than the basis for any "biological" insight on Crocker's part. How could one allow children who were wrecking everything in sight into – of all things – a deep swimming pool? Crocker began to rethink her approach. She knew that certain children were good swimmers so she let them use the pool at their own discretion. But because she was unable to monitor it constantly, she wrote out this permission on slips of paper for every child on an individual basis. It was this practice, she further recalled, that gave rise to the ticket system, which made it possible to record individual patterns of activity – which the two directors later regarded as the results of social syntheses.

The archives contain two letters from Crocker to Scott Williamson of May 1935 that corroborate her recollections. In reading them, however, one feels almost manipulated into believing in a specific version of the Peckham story. The letters feature Crocker's handwritten marginal notes, clearly added much later, which are meant to elucidate her growing understanding, such as: "Light beginning to dawn", "Floods of light here". In these letters Crocker informed her boss of her efforts to organize activities for the children in order to calm things down at the centre. It had, for example, dawned on her, with hindsight, that it made little sense to keep the children busy in isolation from their parents, as this allowed the latter to remain passive.[17] It is instructive to read these essentially practical ruminations together with correspondence between Scott Williamson and his sister. This was written a few months later, in August 1935, and is in the same file. It reveals what Crocker was trying to achieve in her auto-commentary: she appears to have calibrated her assessments *ex post* with far more fundamental ideas held by Scott Williamson, which the latter set out to his sister. Edith Scott Williamson was herself a doctor – and gravely disappointed. Her brother, she averred, had created a truly impressive building. But the whole thing was "lost, rudderless"; it had "no soul, no direction", as she wrote to him. The centre was full of beer-drinking mothers and roistering children; everywhere one looked there were piles of dirty dishes:

> I think it is the human element that is at fault. [...] You are either understaffed, or your staff is bad. There should be a daily inspection; half an hour would do it by someone in authority. Dirt and destruction will wreck your scheme.[18]

Scott Williamson, she asserted, must end this state of affairs so he could devote himself entirely to his medical research. However, his reply reveals that by now he was barely concerned with medicine:

> You are right in all your criticisms. If I were shaping the new world on the basis of the old, I'd do just as you advise: I would "Establish Authority" with a Big Stick. [...] It is the way of Soviets, Hitlers and Mussolinis and our own lesser SHMO [Senior Hospital Medical Officers].[19]

But, he went on, "[o]ur discoveries – if they are discoveries – point to responbility [sic] as the Biological Characteristic of Organism. Authority and responsibility are mutually antipathetic". The priority, then, was not simply to combat authority. A crucial phrase captured his real goal: "enlisting nature [...] on my side." Scott Williamson concluded: "There is both discipline and system in Authority – oh yes! But there is No order. I don't want Machine-made men, or Barrack-made; I am looking for World-made men, natural men." Clean cups, Scott Williamson believed, could provide no shortcut to order. His "distant vision" allowed him no time to concern himself with dirty feet; what was at stake here was nothing less than a rebirth: "[I]t looks ugly – so do all new births." It seems – not long after the opening of the new centre – that Scott Williamson had an at least visionary inkling of the self-organizing capacity of human "nature", which could emerge from specific conditions of empowerment. He took up his sister's nautical metaphor, turning it into a positive: rather than being off-course, the project was an "expedition" into the unknown.[20]

While this may seem prophetic, it should not be overlooked that there is a reason why Crocker's and Scott Williamson's letters are to be found in the same folder. The file was created only in the 1970s when work began on *The Quality of Life*. It is the product of later attempts to make sense of the experiment. Pearse even had Scott Williamson's letter to his sister reprinted in her book, as if to demonstrate that he was right all along to reject intervention at the centre. Because in a chapter entitled "Out of Chaos" she went on to depict how the problems abated after a few months: the first clubs formed quite spontaneously, enhancing the "richness of the social milieu" as a whole and, above all, prompting the children to engage in less destructive activities.[21] Little by little an "orderly 'calm'" had emerged, partly because users were informed of the results of the initial examinations. The chaos of the first few months, which the researchers initially preferred to hush up, had now come to play an argumentational role. For Pearse, sometime between 1935 and 1936 life itself had made its presence felt at the centre. A "bionomic" order, she wrote, had taken hold.[22] The chaos could now be interpreted as birth pangs. At the same time it served as a badge of integrity, as evidence of a determination to resist the impulse to intervene and impose order, which would have distorted the scientific findings.

Mary Langman's recollections

Interestingly, not everyone involved in the experiment saw it that way. Shortly after Pearse's death in 1978 a number of former staff members began to discuss how they might present "Peckham" as cohesively as possible. Around this time they were trying to get new versions of the centre off the ground in a variety of locations, which required negotiations with financial backers and other relevant parties.[23] Douglas Trotter, who had taken over Crocker's role as curator after the war,[24] set himself up as historian of the project. He began to amass former staff members' reminiscences. It soon became clear that Mary Langman, personal assistant to both directors in the 1930s and 1940s, held a dissonant view of the nature, cause and sequence of events during the first few years. Langman did not deny that the centre was an astonishingly harmonious place. In her opinion, however, the reason for this was a complicated "virtuous circle" that hardly confirmed Scott Williamson's and Pearse's biological theories. As Langman saw it, the crucial factors were Scott Williamson's friendly, informal habitus and – even more important – the presence of Jack Donaldson, who had taken on a wide variety of tasks at the centre on a voluntary basis in the 1930s. The way they dealt with members, she contended, was refreshingly different from other social workers' condescending approach:

> Dod and Jack were able to create an atmosphere of trust and confidence in which people felt free to respond in completely new ways. Here nobody was trying to exploit them, or to "get at them", or even "improve" them and do them good.[25]

But Langman also underlined that it was some of the first members themselves who had actively brought the idea of allowing users to organize activities into play not long after the centre opened. In a letter to Trotter from 1983 she emphasized that Donaldson in particular had enjoyed members' trust because he had responded by sitting down with them and discussing how they might best self-administer their clubs.[26]

Pearse and Scott Williamson regarded the users of their centre as manifestations of their biological potential; Langman, meanwhile, called them by name. She praised the colourful owner of a betting shop, Bill Dannan, who founded the centre's much-loved dance band shortly after it opened. A Mr Stockwell had asked for permission to establish a billiards club, which was open to beginners. Langman also recalled a factory owner who responded to one of his workers greeting him at the centre as "sir" by stating: "that won't do here." And she mentioned a "convinced Marxist, who against all theory accepted that Dod and Jack were acting in a way that was in no way inspired by their class interest".[27] Looking back, Langman did not see life itself at work but rather a constellation of individuals thrown together by happy coincidence:

> It is misleading to write that this [order] came about for the negative reason that the staff organised nothing, so that they [the members] were left to get on with it. [T]he old habits that were shed in the Centre were largely class attitudes [...]. [T]hat in pre-war England, with a membership that ranged from doctors to dustmen, "class" differences never proved divisive or embarrassing, really is remarkable.[28]

Elsewhere Langman conjectured that the somewhat chaotic conditions had in fact only come about because Scott Williamson, who had already developed his first theories on the natural order by the mid 1930s, failed to impart them effectively. Rather than providing the staff with consistent instructions, he constantly improvised: "[T]he 'chaos' was not all due to apathetic and bewildered members, but also to bewildered staff, who were told to stop doing what they had been engaged to, but not what they should do."[29] A few years earlier, Crocker too had remarked that with little to do, during the first few months the swimming and gymnastics teachers wandered through the building trying to restrain the children, often banning them from the building. For the most part Pearse and Scott Williamson immediately revoked these bans. Some employees, according to Crocker, were then subject to outright bullying.[30]

Revisions: "socialized science"

What are we to make of these versions of the Peckham story? Had the spontaneous social order, which the centre researchers soon began to interpret as a biological fact, always been there, waiting to be discovered? Did the medical directors actually impede its development through their inconsistently implemented rules? And was the "chaos" really brought to an end when certain users and staff members put their heads together? Significantly, three years after the centre's inauguration, some employees still wanted to see a crackdown.[31] It appears that, rather than every problem being decisively resolved, what we can discern here is a learning process, as a result of which at least some of those involved no longer defined certain conditions as chaos.

This is what emerges from the second, shortest (and least-cited) book by Pearse and Scott Williamson, which appeared in 1938: *Biologists in Search of Material. An Interim Report on the Work of the Pioneer Health Centre.* When it comes to the presentation of medical findings it differs little from *The Peckham Experiment.* In contrast to its successor, however, the book does not limit itself to successes. In fact, here Pearse and Scott Williamson concede that the search for "material" had been more difficult than initially expected. The centre had come nowhere near to attracting the number of members they had literally counted on in order to cover its financial needs. It could cater to a maximum of 2,000 families but had never got beyond just over 700, many of whom, moreover, failed to renew their membership each week. Pearse and Scott Williamson explained that Peckham residents' evident disinterest had opened their eyes to people's resistance to being improved in accordance with "outside standards".[32] They wrote:

> Our failures during our first eighteen months' work have taught us something very significant. Individuals, from infants to old people, resent or fail to show any interest in anything initially presented to them through discipline, regulation or instruction which is another aspect of authority. (Even the very "Centre idea" has a certain taint of authority and this is contributing to our slow recruitment.)[33]

Any attempt to make people change their way of life must therefore be avoided if there is to be any hope of getting at the "source and origin of spontaneous action". "We now proceed by merely providing an environment rich in instruments for action." This, we are told, had not only eliminated the chaos that initially marred everyday life at the centre. It had also fostered Peckham residents' interest in the experiment. (This is something the text implies rather than proving with the aid of higher membership figures.) For our authors, then, "Peckham" was also instructive as a study of methods: "As one of our colleagues remarked – it seems that 'a sort of anarchy' is the first condition in any experiment in human applied biology."[34]

The advertising brochures that continued to be sent out to potential members in the district bear witness to the pair's new insight. From 1936 on, these publications no longer highlighted just medical services and leisure activities but also users' opportunities to contribute to life and research at the centre. One leaflet stated: "We want you to form the Club and run it yourselves, for yourselves."[35] Another concludes as follows: "You have the chance to co-operate in this great experiment. [...] You have the chance to influence it, to make it grow in the right way. Why not come in and see what you're missing?"[36]

Hence, the clearer it became that the Peckham researchers themselves were an obstacle to the unfolding of "biological" self-organization, the more it appears to have come to the fore as an object of study. Of necessity, Pearse and Scott Williamson continued, they had imposed on themselves the very discipline that was hampering users' participation in the experiment: "We have had to learn to sit back and wait for these activities to emerge. [...] [W]e have had to cultivate more and more patience in ourselves."[37]

It was not entirely honest then, that by 1943 Pearse was reinterpreting as a *prerequisite* for scientific research what she and Scott Williamson had presented just a few years earlier as the *result* of piecemeal modifications of the laboratory. Most commentators now portrayed the experiment as an attempt to verify a clearly defined thesis and test out an equally well thought-through methodology. *The Peckham Experiment* asks, though only rhetorically:

[H]ow can such an unfamiliar and objective factor as the scientist and observer be introduced into any social milieu without instantly shattering its spontaneity? The answer seems to lie in the possibility that the scientist himself and his technicians should become one of the accepted groups forming the cultural diversity in the environment.[38]

More and more often, texts by the Peckham directors now discussed, albeit metaphorically, this "participant observation" at the centre.[39] Here they tended to evoke nautical imagery, referring to dives and voyages. The building was often described as a ship while the research project was conceptualized as an expedition without a compass, a metaphor deployed by Scott Williamson as early as 1936. Life at the centre, *The Peckham Experiment* tells us, may be described as a matter of give and take, an "open field upon which every influence may play free as the changing winds, [...] the observers themselves being of the company and functioning in unity with the whole". Researchers and users both dived into a "pool of information"; at the centre knowledge was distributed in every direction: "[A] continuous trickle of [...] facts flows throughout the whole Centre organisation, tending – like any fluid – to spread gradually over the whole field."[40] If we recall the clear boundaries between workers and their educators that pervaded texts written in the early 1930s, it is remarkable that *The Peckham Experiment* states:

[At] the end of four years there is little to distinguish members from staff in the social interplay of the Centre. The whole medium is social – Science socialised. The Centre has, in fact, shown itself to be a potent mechanism for the "democratisation" of knowledge and action.[41]

As mentioned earlier, in retrospect Pearse and Crocker described the centre building as a significant component of this democratizing mechanism. One could see through the glass walls, "as the cytologist may under his microscope watch living cells grow out in a culture medium", as they stated in 1943.[42]

Later, Pearse went so far as to stylize the building as a "bioscope", an optical instrument that had made it possible to observe life itself.[43] Above all, though, the Peckham researchers were soon asserting that, in collaboration with architect Owen Williams, Scott Williamson had consciously designed the building in such a way as to turn all those involved into researchers: "With no embarrassing thresholds to cross, there will be no exclusive groups and no intimidating hierarchies."[44]

Nonetheless, laws both written and unwritten continued to apply. Pearse and Crocker mentioned, for example, though only in passing, that access to the swimming pool was controlled, that someone checked whether children could swim a whole length in the small pool before they were allowed to use the large one, and that efforts were made to ensure that users took off their outdoor shoes before entering the gymnasium.[45] A large sign near the edge of the pool declared that each user was permitted to stay in the water for just one and a half hours at a time, with a bell marking its passage.[46] Above all, however, at no point was users' self-administration of the centre as a whole subject to debate, not even the possibility of giving them a say on the use of their membership fees or the membership criteria.

Genius and autocrat

Overall it seems that clear rules had been superseded by Scott Williamson's benign authority. In her memoirs Frances Donaldson characterized him as follows:

> [H]e was not interested in how people should behave, or in how they might be made to behave, but only in how they did behave in any given circumstances. He was accused often [...] of lacking the scientific mind, because he could never be induced to conduct his experiment on the lines and with the methods which other people thought necessary if results were to have a widespread effect. But in his dealing with people he had an objectivity that was almost inhuman. And this made for the kind of democracy in the Centre which I doubt has ever been seen anywhere else. He used to walk about the social floors observing the members, and only when he noted that some thread of behaviour was upsetting the pattern of natural response to opportunity of the mass of the people did he move to control it.[47]

This passage gives us an idea of how the observation of social order at the centre proceeded in the late 1930s. It was Scott Williamson himself who strolled through the building, manufacturing many of the behavioural patterns the researchers sought to observe. Apparently, the preconditions for the biological order that had just been discovered had to be actively maintained. Yet only Scott Williamson seems to have had the gift for defining where this order turned into its opposite, as Donaldson hints. He made corrections to group activities whenever he believed they were showing signs of over-organization or exclusivity. He appears to have taken users convicted of such misconduct to task in his characteristically friendly way. Some clubs, such as the advanced billiards group, he relegated to smaller rooms so as not to put off potential imitators. In Peckham, then, paradoxically, freedom from authority was established unsystematically and by fiat. The PHC was governed by an autocrat despite the fact such figures were Scott Williamson's declared enemy, if we are to believe Donaldson:

> He had a rooted objection to the leader in society, as someone who pushed around the human material he wished to study in spontaneous action, and who exerted the force of his personality to drive more ordinary people out of the rut of their natural behaviour into activities unsuited to them and which they half-consciously disliked.[48]

Donaldson, however, does not explain how a man who spoke out against every form of external influence could simultaneously be characterized as follows:

> He was a dictator; a benevolent, sweet tempered, untyrannical dictator, but still a dictator. He refused at all times to act except in the light of his own vision, and he could not be moved to any form of compromise with the ideas of other people.[49]

Time and again the General Committee, which according to the centre's statutes had the last word on its fate, had to rubberstamp decisions already implemented by Scott Williamson. In view of such arbitrary acts it comes as no surprise that Donaldson describes her colleagues as disciples, even as "voluntary guinea-pigs, because of their belief in the genius of this man".[50] By the mid 1930s Scott Williamson had created a setting in which his charisma could effloresce. Before members of the London Anarchist Group – of all people – he even made a statement that would seem like a bon mot had he not been quite serious: "I was the only person with authority and I used it to stop anyone exerting any authority."[51]

Most of those involved in the centre, it must be said, were entirely content with this situation. The archives contain numerous photos of festivities at the centre, and while they show lively scenes they also reveal hierarchies. Here Scott Williamson – his authority undiminished by a cardboard party hat – always occupies a central position.[52] A pencil drawing has also survived showing him as a giant, pontificating with index finger raised amid a group of devoted listeners.[53]

It is now becoming clear why no truly consistent method was ever developed at the centre. Scott Williamson had the final say. His colleagues were instructed to inform him of every observation they thought important, often doing so in the cafeteria, where they tended to congregate towards evening.[54] Scott Williamson liked to think out loud and walks through the building with colleagues provided another arena for the development of his ideas.[55] To all appearances he used their observations in a highly selective way, though he showed little interest in scrutinizing them. In the 1970s Lucy Crocker recalled:

> [I]n the centre I frequently told him of something that I had observed (which he certainly hadn't seen in such detail and which he immediately accepted) and within hours or days had incorporated into his writing or discussions.[56]

She added: "He seemed to me to be moving in the centre in a totally digestive and creative relationship with his environmental threshold – the members." Scott Williamson's interpretive monopoly, then, was partly due to his seeming embodiment of the centre's modus operandi. More than anyone else, he had mastered the art of creative synthesis with his objects of study. As his colleagues saw it, he was a man who knew how to make highly efficient use of his environment. At the same time he continually enriched it by disseminating his insights in an attempt to expedite the quasi-evolutionary process of cooperation between people at various stages of development.

The biologist as the summit of creation

Shortly after the centre got up and running Scott Williamson began to organize intermittent, so-called "Sunday meetings", which, it should be noted, were entirely non-religious, unlike similar events in the settlement houses of the nineteenth century. He kicked off the first of these meetings in February 1936 by reporting that many members had asked him about the purpose of the experiment. The answer, he stated, was straightforward. The users provided the researchers with "material (your own lives) for observation and experiment". He added: "[W]e find it unnecessary to tell you what you *ought* to do."[57] According to Scott Williamson, it was users' "common sense" that kept the centre going. "[I]t is no longer we doctors and the Centre staff who are running the Centre. You members are carrying out this experiment in what life is and how it may be lived."[58] Nonetheless Scott Williamson then went on to present an initial premise. The family, he explained, is the basic unit of organic life because it induces altruism, and this is of fundamental importance to society: "[T]he biological attribute of altruism becomes more necessary, to prevent the world going to pieces through egoism." He concluded by emphasizing to his listeners: "These things should thread through your minds."[59]

A few months later Scott Williamson began his next lecture as follows: "The last Sunday meeting you remember, we formed ourselves into a band of Pioneers."[60] He reminded his listeners of the numerous visitors who had come to the centre over the last few weeks. While they had been a source of disruption, their interest in the centre was understandable. They were in search of "knowledge, information [...] on dealing with the great social problems which face the world".[61] He went on:

> [I]n joining the Centre you have become serious partners in a team of research workers. It is my misfortune and responsibility to be No. 1 in this research team, and No. 1 in a research team does not mean anything personal, nor does it mean that you all have to follow me, but it does mean that you have all to catch something of the knowledge that Dr. Pearse and I have acquired during the course of the experiment. It is not enough to like us and trust us, you have to try and understand the scientist's point of view. Somehow or other you have to try and become an active member of the team and being so you are as responsible as any other part of a whole body.

Scott Williamson, as clearly evident in the typescript of his presentation, saw himself as the head of the organic community of researchers he had forged in the previous meeting. But it is also apparent that he improvised from one talk to the next:

> Now the first Sunday meeting led me to think that I was not playing quite fair with my fellow workers: That I had a lot of information and tit bits up my sleeve, which were not being produced. Even the staff blame me at times for keeping them in the dark![62]

As if to legitimize this knowledge gap he now described the evolution of the human brain, culminating in the capacity for rational thought, which had superseded intuition: scientists, he contended, were seekers after truth, with no interest in intervention: "[A] sort of abstract individual, he [the scientist] does not want to manipulate things." This, he went on, had made scientists into observers who had investigated the physical world in detail. In doing so, they had for a while lost their capacity to analyse wholes. But now they had reached the next stage: *biologists* were beginning to study life itself.[63] Scott Williamson clearly regarded individuals capable of carrying out such holistic research as the peak of natural human development. His talks, accordingly, increasingly revolved around his own activities. The final surviving typescript is entitled: "What sort of man is a scientist?" It is exceedingly muddled. It would be good, to cite the core message, if more people looked at the world as scientists do, but they should investigate not just facts but "facts in action". Yet Scott Williamson also warned his listeners that: "[D]efinitions are very misleading things."[64] At the Sunday meetings Scott Williamson thus linked the imperative of getting involved in the experiment with the greatest of moral responsibilities: solving the social problems of the modern world. But he left open the crucial question of how precisely one ought to carry out research. The main thing was *that* such research was done – by every single member of the community.

Notes

1 Annual Report 1936, WL, SA/PHC/A.2/9, 8.
2 These pre-printed forms were drawn up by Scott Williamson's brother Bruce, who was also a doctor: WL, SA/PHC/D.1/14.
3 See the documents in WL, SA/PHC/B.3/3.
4 There were 27 individuals working at the PHC in 1948, from the directors to the cleaners. Evidently, lists were produced because at this time the personnel was subject to a high degree of fluctuation. But they had also become necessary due to Pearse's and Scott Williamson's lengthy periods of absence (for lecture tours).
5 Medical Department, May 1948, WL, SA/PHC/B.5/5/1.
6 Reception Desk: appointments system etc., c. 1948, WL, SA/PHC/B.5/5/2.
7 Ibid.
8 Social Floor, August 1948, WL, SA/PHC/B.5/5/3.
9 Stallibrass, *The Self-Respecting Child*, 24–25.
10 Planned since 1938, prior to the war the keys proved too costly and could not be implemented after it due to copper rationing (The "Centre Key", 1938, WL, SA/PHC/B.3/6), while the plans drawn up by Bell Telephones to develop a device to record the family consultation also came to nothing: Pearse, *The Quality of Life*, 87. In view of the failure to introduce them, David Armstrong's interpretation of the keys as the paradigmatic tool of an all-controlling "medical gaze" seems overblown: David Armstrong, "The Rise of Surveillance Medicine", *Sociology of Health & Illness* 17, no. 3 (1995): 398.
11 In 1950, at a time when the centre had been shut down and its members were pulling out all the stops to get it reopened, they went so far as to approach a number of MPs (see Chapter 10). Elsie Purser, spokesperson for the users' delegation, was asked: "How is it actually run?" Purser referred to extensive self-administration by users. When asked more specifically about the scientific practices deployed, her answer seemed more straightforward, but in fact leaves us none the wiser: "Q: Did the Doctors stand around with notebooks in their hands? A. (There was great merriment among the delegation at this mental picture) I had hardly any need to answer NO" (minutes of meeting, March 23, 1950, WL, SA/PHC/B.6/4). Notes are cited in just one location, in Stallibrass's book. With respect to "22.1." and the four-year-old "Brian O.", we are informed that the latter rapidly taught himself how to use roller-skates (Stallibrass, *The Self-Respecting Child*, 22). This scenario is also paraphrased in *The Peckham Experiment*, supplemented by the claim that a hundred other examples could be given (Pearse and Crocker, *The Peckham Experiment*, 201). Adge Elven, assistant to the curator after the war, recalled in 1984 that he noted down individual patterns, furnishing them with little symbols for different activities – whether with the help of tickets or on the basis of personal observations is unclear: Reminiscences of St Mary's Road Peckham, June/October 1984, WL, SA/PHC/C.20, 13.
12 Staff list, 1934, WL, SA/PHC/A.1/3.
13 Pearse, *The Quality of Life*, 25–26.
14 Pearse to Crocker, January 25, 1970, WL, SA/PHC/E.15/1. Crocker had got married and was now called Pearce, but given the risk of confusing her with Innes Pearse I will continue to use her maiden name.
15 Lucy Pearce, Chaos in the Centre. Notes on Children (1935–36), 1970, WL, SA/PHC/E.15/1, 2.
16 Ibid., 3.
17 Crocker to Scott Williamson, May 30, 1935, WL, SA/PHC/B.3/7/1–2.
18 Edith to George Scott Williamson [August 1935], WL, SA/PHC/B.3/7/3–4.
19 George to Edith Scott Williamson [August 1935], WL, SA/PHC/B.3/7/3–4.
20 All quotes: ibid.

21 Pearse, *The Quality of Life*, 27–28, 35.
22 Ibid., 143.
23 See Chapter 11.
24 He was apparently sent to London by George MacLeod, founder of the ecumenical Iona Community in Scotland.
25 Mary Langman, Social Development [early 1980s], WL, SA/PHC/C.13, 2.
26 Langman to Trotter, June 22, 1983, WL, SA/PHC/C.13.
27 Mary Langman, Social Development, WL, SA/PHC/C.13, 2.
28 Ibid.
29 The Peckham Experiment, Tape 2, undated, [c. 1983], WL, SA/PHC/C.13, 2.
30 Lucy Pearce, Chaos in the Centre. Notes on Children (1935–36), 1970, WL, SA/PHC/E.15/1, 3. Just a few members of staff, according to Langman, managed to deal creatively with the new situation, including one female colleague "who was inspired to invent a game in the gym which eventually led to the 'freegym' described in 'the P. Expt'". In passing, then, we learn that the children's anarchical-harmonious swinging in the gymnasium was something the staff had come up with. Langman to Trotter, June 22, 1983, WL, SA/PHC/C.13.
31 Minutes, Executive Committee, November 30, 1938, WL, SA/PHC/A.1/4.
32 Scott Williamson and Pearse, *Biologists in Search of Material*, 38.
33 Ibid.
34 Ibid., 38–40.
35 What the Centre is, undated [c. 1937], WL, SA/PHC/B.3/22/2.
36 The Centre, St Mary's Road, Peckham, SE15, undated [c. 1937], WL, SA/PHC/B.3/22/1.
37 Scott Williamson and Pearse, *Biologists in Search of Material*, 38.
38 Pearse and Crocker, *The Peckham Experiment*, 46–47.
39 Pearse and Scott Williamson did not use this term itself; in general they neglected to follow the methodological debates in ethnology and social anthropology. Yet participant observation was already subject to initial efforts at formalization in the 1930s, at the LSE as elsewhere, including with respect to the study of induced behaviour in so-called field experiments.
40 Pearse and Crocker, *The Peckham Experiment*, 48, 79, 92. The reader too was urged to forget his pre-existing knowledge: "[P]repared to sail upon the open sea of humanity where the manifold winds of the environment play in ceaseless change, he may set out on a further search into the science of Living [sic]." Ibid., 26.
41 Ibid., 78.
42 Ibid., 241.
43 Pearse, *The Quality of Life*, 12.
44 "The Open Door", *Peckham*, September/October 1949, 7, WL, SA/PHC/B.5/22 (also available at "Peckham and Architecture. A drama of building and people", www.sochealth.co.uk/1949/09/21/peckham/ (accessed December 17, 2017)). Tellingly, the architect of the building was far from pleased with this version of its history, which pre-empted the more recent interpretation outlined in the introduction. Williams demanded a correction. He had, he asserted, designed the building on St Mary's Road all by himself. Williams to Scott Williamson, October 19, 1949, WL, SA/PHC/B.5/13/3.
45 Pearse and Crocker, *The Peckham Experiment*, 190–191.
46 Long Room, c. 1920s–1930s, WL, SA/PHC/H.1/16.
47 Donaldson, *Child of the Twenties*, 159.
48 Ibid., 160.
49 Ibid., 163.
50 Ibid., 159. Their temporary cohabitation and "romantic idealism" went too far for her taste; ibid., 164–165.
51 Quoted in: Ward, "A Laboratory of Anarchy", 60.

52 Parties, c. 1920s–1930s, WL, SA/PHC/H.1/14.
53 Pencil sketch of GSW, "The Great Man with his people", 1938, WL, SA/PHC/D.1/5.
54 Alison Stallibrass, *Being Me and Also Us. Lessons from the Peckham Experiment* (Edinburgh: Scottish Academic Press, 1989), 129.
55 Donaldson, *Child of the Twenties*, 161.
56 Pearce, addressee unclear, undated [1970s], WL, SA/PHC/E.3/112–114.
57 G. S. W. First Sunday Meeting, February 16, 1936, WL, SA/PHC/B.3a/9, 1 (original emphasis).
58 Ibid., 2.
59 Ibid., 3–4.
60 Typescript of lecture, undated [September 1936], WL, SA/PHC/B.3a/9, 1.
61 Ibid.
62 Ibid., 2
63 Ibid., 2.
64 Typescript of lecture, undated [1936/37], WL, SA/PHC/B.3/9, 2, 3.

6　Interim findings

The Pioneer Health Centre on St Mary's Road was intended to flesh out the conclusions reached during the pilot project on Queen's Road: the best way to induce individuals to take responsibility for their health was to facilitate their self-initiated adaption of knowledge, which must be freely available in an informal, everyday situation. In their focus on identifying the best means to activate a personal sense of responsibility, which included attention to the needs of one's nearest and dearest, the founders of the PHC shared the goals of older, indeed Victorian theories of social work. They also echoed nineteenth-century reformers' belief that the best way to remedy social hardships was to help people help themselves on a case-by-case basis.

However, during the planning of the new centre this belief was fused with a scientific aspiration introduced mainly by doctors Pearse and Scott Williamson. Having initially only joined the project to evaluate its success through follow-up medical examinations, the two doctors began to turn a project of reform into a research project. As designated medical directors they sought to achieve a different, more neutral approach to the objects of their research: the centre's members. Pearse and Scott Williamson asked themselves how, in their new laboratory, they themselves could avoid disrupting the spontaneous exchange of information between its users. Before the centre had opened, then, they did at least intend to rid themselves of an urge to intervene when confronted with untreated illnesses and unhealthy habits. Accordingly, they saw themselves less as active educators and more as a passive knowledge resource for the centre's future members.

Not long after the inauguration of the new building, in the summer of 1935, this hands-off attitude became even more important, but for reasons the medical directors had not previously anticipated: the human "material" failed to accumulate by itself on the scale expected – a particularly thorny problem in economic terms, as the lack of membership fees was threatening to scupper the costly project. The new members, moreover, failed to take advantage of many of the social and sporting options at the centre. Its operators were soon putting both things down to users being put off by excessive organization, by too many rules and timetables. A cumulative pressure thus arose to extend members' freedoms, or to put it differently, to limit the options for sanctioning them, particularly among the lower-ranking staff. Centre employees were enjoined to practise passivity in the face of improper use of sporting equipment and furnishings and cavorting children. Once implemented, it was near-impossible to rescind this decision, in part because the centre directors were now trying to make membership palatable to potential local users by highlighting the freedoms they would enjoy there. Certain individuals such as Lucy Crocker and Jack Donaldson – probably frustrated by unclear instructions – began to experiment with the administration of the leisure activities at the centre in cooperation with certain users. The rules were enforced with ever less stringency.

In parallel to this, Scott Williamson appears to have extended his ideas on the natural foundation of "respons-ability", which he had already developed by the early 1930s, to the social interplay at the centre. He regarded the fact that some members got involved in the first self-administered clubs as confirmation of these ideas and he now began to provide his colleagues' restrained approach to members with a theoretical foundation. A cross-section of the publications by Scott Williamson, Pearse and Lucy Crocker reveals that they gradually reinterpreted the centre as a place where it was possible to study the "*living structure of society*" per se. A means to an end – the wide range of activities from which centre users could choose was intended to help expedite their journey towards health – became an end in itself as these researchers observed the effects of this freedom, which they now equated with "health" or "life". Sometime between 1935 and 1939, then, a medical field experiment turned into a sociobiological one.

The architecture of the centre, too, appears to have played a role in this reinterpretation. At the very least, its flexible, transparent ground plan presented no obstacle to intensifying contact with users, in order, if desired, to impart knowledge to them and observe the results of this inculcation at close range. The researchers' own daily interactions with the residents of Peckham, who could largely do as they wished, likely made them even more receptive to the advantages of spontaneous human interaction.

But more crucial to this receptivity were the holistic grand theories that Scott Williamson and Pearse projected onto the social processes at the centre. Prompted by the findings of evolutionary biology and reform eugenics, histology and nutritional science, as they were circulating in progressive academic circles in Britain in the 1930s, they interpreted the interpersonal stimulation observed at the centre as the cumulative enrichment of an environment with socio-metabolic products. In fact, the centre seemed to suggest how one might cultivate the species itself, nudging it onto a natural upward trajectory. This naturalization, however, made the social problems that had motivated the establishment of the first centre in the mid 1920s seem ever more secondary. As they came to regard human interactions as processes of synthesis between biological entities, the researchers at the centre lost sight of the social status of Peckham's residents, who were transformed from exponents of the urban working classes into a representative sample of humanity itself.

Hence, the specific – epistemological, social, economic and architectural – situation in which the centre's directors, curators and their assistants found themselves in the mid 1930s sensitized them to social microprocesses. Under Scott Williamson's affable and charismatic tutelage, everywhere they looked his colleagues began to discern interactions between individual patterns of activity with positive effects on life at the centre as a whole.[1] Furthermore, the border-crossing interactions within the centre that had now become manifest resulted in a modified evaluation of scientific routes to generating knowledge. When the researchers came face to face with the living data they were observing, lived experience and scientific discovery became ever harder to tell apart. The Peckham experience became a significant part of the Peckham Experiment.[2] This made those studied in the experiment seem less like objects and more like partners in a particularly democratic research project. And it allowed the directors to set off in search of new, qualitative ways of lending their work plausibility.

Any attempt at reconstructing the events of the Peckham Experiment is thus hampered by the reinterpretations bound up with this development, the often unacknowledged learning processes and the operators' shifting nomenclature, not to mention their outright romanticization of everyday life at the centre. Former staff members faced the same problem as they struggled to agree on a single version of the project's history in the 1970s and 1980s. It is ultimately impossible to pin down one reality of the Peckham Experiment, in part because the insights the researchers took from it were continually fed back into the centre community in order to stimulate its growth. As a result, multiple meanings were attached to the centre. This will become clear in the following chapters, which turn to the traces left behind by centre users. One chapter deals with photographs from the centre, another with the recollections and publications of its members – the guinea pigs, as some of them referred to themselves. Both chapters seek, from a micro-historical vantage point, to shed light on the subtle but complex power relations that pervaded the centre, particularly in the post-war period, before the second part of the book resumes its earlier chronology.

Notes

1 Douglas Trotter recalled in 1984 that he had learned to see "patterns" when he observed families: Reminiscences of St Mary's Road Peckham, June/October 1984, WL, SA/PHC/C.20.
2 As affirmed by Alison Stallibrass, The Peckham Experience; A hope for a healthier future, 1984, WL, SA/PHC/C.18/5.

7 The centre in photographs
Visual stimulation and participant observation

Many accounts that seek to recall the positive lessons of the Peckham Experiment base themselves on photographs of everyday life at the St Mary's Road centre. Life at the Pioneer Health Centre does in fact make an unorganized impression in these photos. There is, for example, little sign of the infamous mass ornaments described by Siegfried Kracauer: images of synchronized bodies, lined up in rows and/or practising gymnastics, which served to visualize healthy, vigorous collectives in many countries in the 1930s. In contrast, many photos from the centre show postures that seem anything but disciplined. The people in them are often laughing and dancing or even dressed up in party attire. This makes it all the more crucial to bear in mind that most of these photographs were intended for public relations work. They do not convey a clear impression of the laboratory conditions in Peckham but are instead interpretations of these conditions. They cannot be cleanly separated from the ideas found in the books in which they are printed. In fact, while the archives contain a large number of photos from the centre,[1] it is always the same ones that crop up in the publications. The authors consistently disseminated specific images.

There are two crucial factors we must consider if we are tempted to imagine that these official photos give us an undistorted view of past reality. The first is that the mere presence of a photographer in a social space, which, even to those photographed, is distinguished chiefly by its informality, almost inevitably has complex effects. The second is the considerable extent to which these photographs reveal situations of reciprocal observation. They are representative of the natural social contagions at the centre. Hence, they can be understood in part as subtle corroboration of the quasi-participatory research carried out within the Peckham Experiment. This makes it all the more remarkable that the archival material provides no indication of any scientific use (in the narrower sense) of photography as a means of documentation, for example.[2]

Holistic perspectives and visual contagions

As a technical process that isolates snippets of reality, did the centre directors suspect photography of having alienating effects? In any event it is striking that the centre was presented less often by individual photographs than by photo series. This applies in particular to the above-mentioned photographic chapter in *The Peckham Experiment*. [3] This modernistic section of the book, featuring asymmetric page frames and humorous annotations, is structured like a visit to the centre. The latter is introduced by a (written) reference to its special atmosphere; an external view of the building is then followed by photographs that seek to convey the first impression a visitor would have of the interior. The observer is present during an examination; he sees a variety of everyday scenes – overwhelmingly group activities towards the end of the visit, the photographs becoming increasingly detailed. Nearing the end of the series we find more and more individual scenes per page, as if the visitor is beginning to perceive the centre as a whole (Figure 7.1).

Many of the photographs that make up the photo series show complex spatial sequences: groups of people in front of windows, glass dividing walls, and open doors behind which other spaces open up. The centre is staged as a structure that invites the user to engage in movement. While wandering around he may take a variety of individual routes, but these always place the activities of others in his way. We see, for example, two girls in bathing suits, who have evidently just got out of the swimming pool. Through the glass wall that separates the latter from the cafeteria, they are now watching other children playing board games, who proceed unperturbed (Figure 7.2).

The photograph on the cover of the 1949–1950 issue of the centre bulletin, *Peckham*, reverses perspective. While it shows a discrete scene, it also appears to depict a process (Figure 7.3). A boy is in the act of jumping into the pool from the diving board, while being observed by other children, potential imitators, some of them in the water, others (still) in the cafeteria. The transition between the active individuals and onlookers is fluid. Both photographs, then, illustrate the thesis that mutual observation among active individuals has a contagious effect; the photographs seem like snapshots of sparks of activity jumping from one person to another.

Such reciprocal stimulation was possible across generational boundaries, as another photo suggests (Figure 7.4). Strikingly, it shows a camera, implying that the photographer himself is being drawn into the action. We can understand photos like this as an attempt to simultaneously illustrate the researchers' participation in the life of the centre and underline the objectivity of their observations. They show people unfazed by the recording of their actions – whether by a camera or roaming scientists, as it appears.

Another photograph from the series in *The Peckham Experiment* brings out the ambivalence of this peculiar conception of objectivity (Figure 7.5). Captioned with the words "Plenty to watch", with its pronounced vanishing point it compels the observer to adopt the photographer's perspective. Given the doubling of the observer's position, which becomes particularly clear in this picture (here we are looking over the shoulder not just of the children looking on but also of the researchers, who are in turn observing the former), any vantage point objectively detached from what is happening is lost in the depths of the image-space. This is all the more important given that, in all

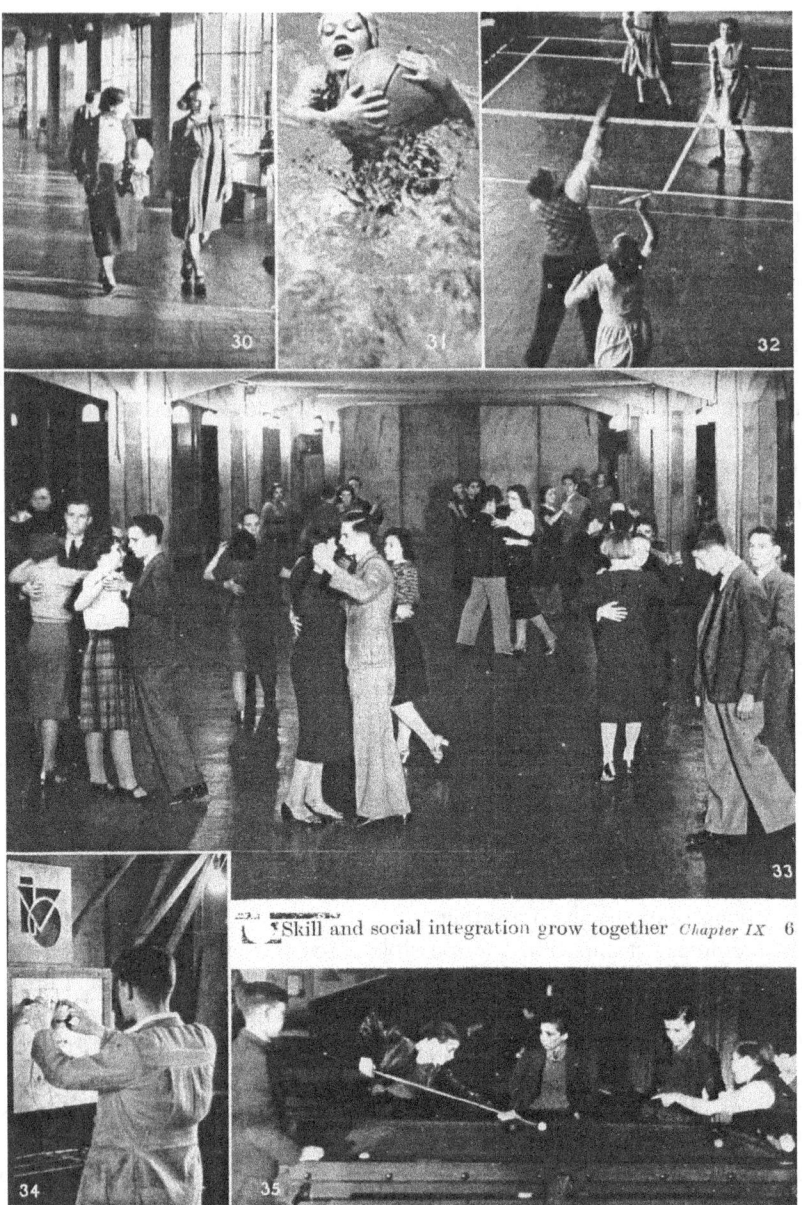

Figure 7.1 A page from the "Chapter in Photographs" captioned "Skill and social integration grow together". The montage of photos of different activities – people dancing, playing darts or badminton, or strolling through the centre – illustrates the diverse range of activities unfolding before the new member's eyes.

(Innes H. Pearse and Lucy H. Crocker, *The Peckham Experiment. A Study of the Living Structure of Society.* London: Allen & Unwin, 1943, 63)

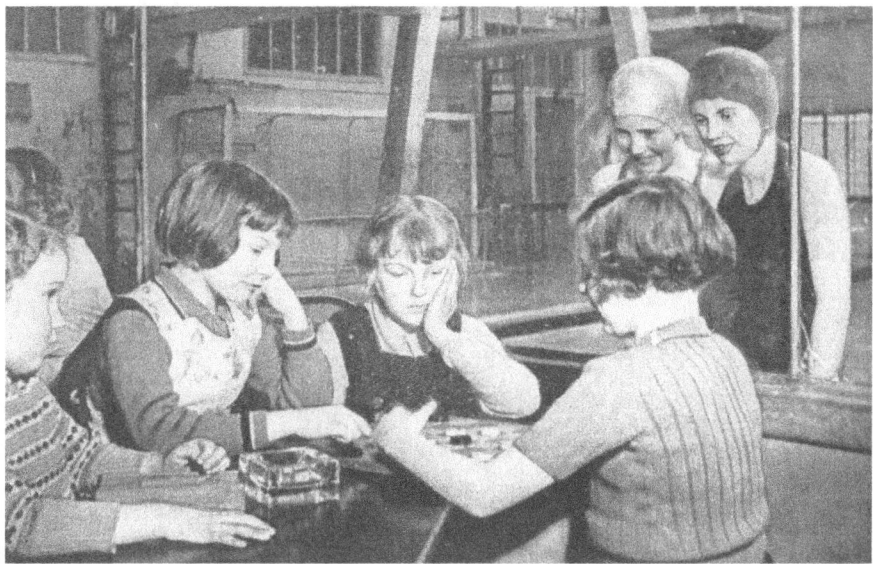

Figure 7.2 Photograph from *The Peckham Experiment*, captioned "Intent on skill ..." (Innes H. Pearse and Lucy H. Crocker, *The Peckham Experiment. A Study of the* Living *Structure of Society*. London: Allen & Unwin, 1943, 62)

likelihood, the authors selected this picture because the children in the fore-ground are marvelling at the epitome of "bionomic" order: rope-swinging in the gymnasium in all its dynamic harmony.

As it happens, as late as 1936, shortly after the centre was opened, a press photo presented the rope-swinging in the gymnasium in a quite different way. Here, the bodies of some female centre members were arranged for the occa-sion. The women in the photograph are all looking towards the photographer, who is unmistakably dominating the proceedings. They look as though they are waiting for a starting signal before becoming active. Here, then, we are not yet dealing with life forging ahead in untrammelled fashion. The same applies to the few published photographs from the original centre on Queen's Road. If centre members appear at all, far from being absorbed in activities they are fully aware they are being photographed. The distinctions between the medical personnel and their beneficiaries are also clearly marked. In one photograph showing the garden on Queen's Road, for example, we see a nurse and, it appears, Scott Williamson, both clad in professional white. Both are standing, framing a group of sitters (Figure 7.6).

Oddly enough there are no photographs at all showing the curators or the medical directors strolling through the centre, with a single exception that I will come to in a moment. Instead, as mentioned earlier, they are shown with the family documents, carrying out examinations and, above all, during the consultations with family members. Here differences between staff members are revealed as well: Pearse and Scott Williamson appear

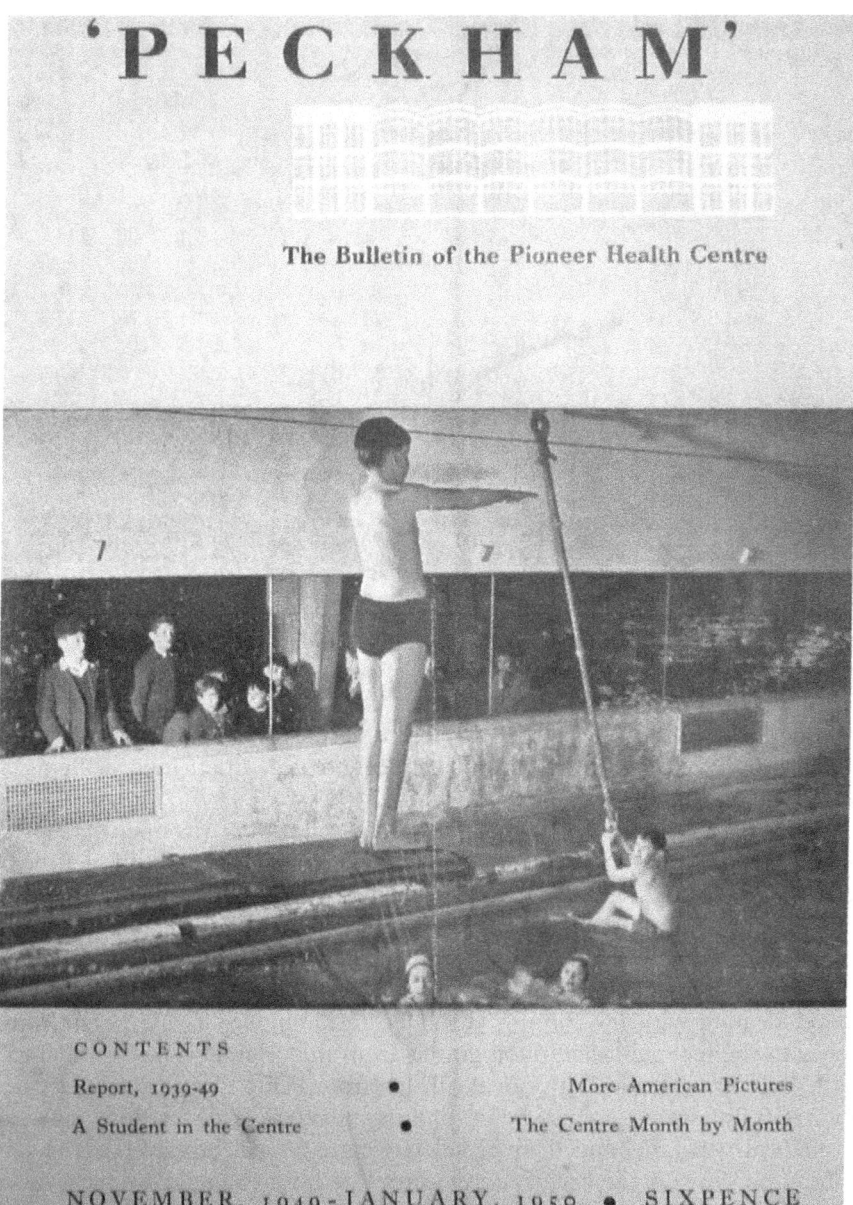

Figure 7.3 One photograph – three stages of social activation
(*Peckham: The Bulletin of the Pioneer Health Centre* (November 1949–January 1950),
WL, SA/PHC/B.5/22, cover image)

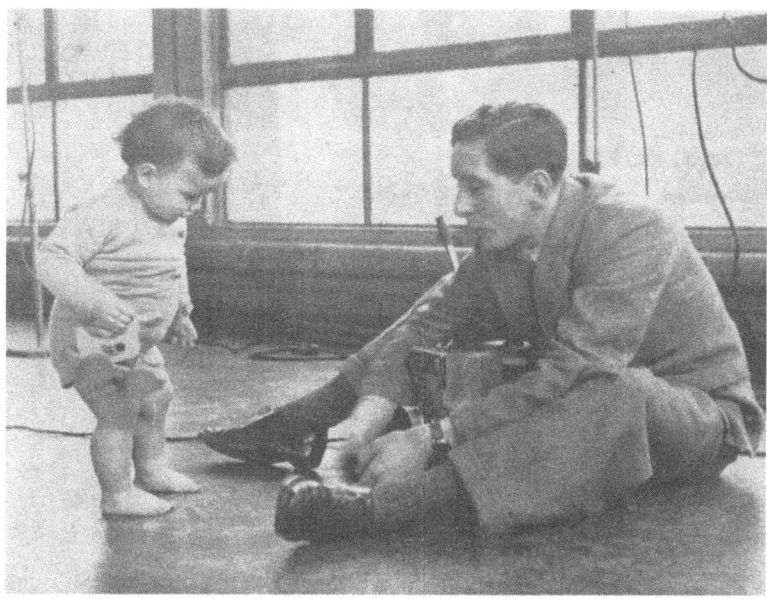

Figure 7.4 "Mutual Observation in the Second Nursery" (1940s)
(Innes H. Pearse, *The Quality of Life: The Peckham Approach to Human Ethology.*
Edinburgh: Scottish Academic Press, 1979, plate 5)

disproportionately often in the printed material on the centre; they alone
represent its scientific aspect. If we take a close look, moreover, we find that
photos showing both biologists and experimental subjects together are
subtly pervaded by power, a power also inherent in the very absence of
authority, manufactured in semi-authoritarian fashion, that we considered
in the previous chapter. However easy-going things may have been, these
photos always reveal asymmetries determining the flow of information. In
one photograph showing a family consultation in the 1940s Scott Williamson is emphasized by an informal but nonetheless elevated sitting posture,
and by the fact that the family are cheerfully listening to his remarks rather
than vice versa (Figure 7.7). It is also clear who has the proverbial last word
on the situation – it is Pearse, in her white lab coat, who is taking the
minutes. Her notebook reminds us of the meta-level of this chat: it was
always subject to observation.

Again, the photo captioned "Mother has a question" does not simply show
a friendly conversation, even if it does in fact record one (Figure 7.8). It was
selected for a publication on the Peckham Experiment because it appears to
exemplify its thesis. Here, someone has learned to seek out knowledge in a
self-responsible way. In reality the title ought to be: "Doctor Pearse gives an
answer": once again in the expert's neutral white, she is dispensing advice to a
depersonalized "mother". There are good reasons why the latter's enquiring
facial expression resembles that of her infant: both mother and child are

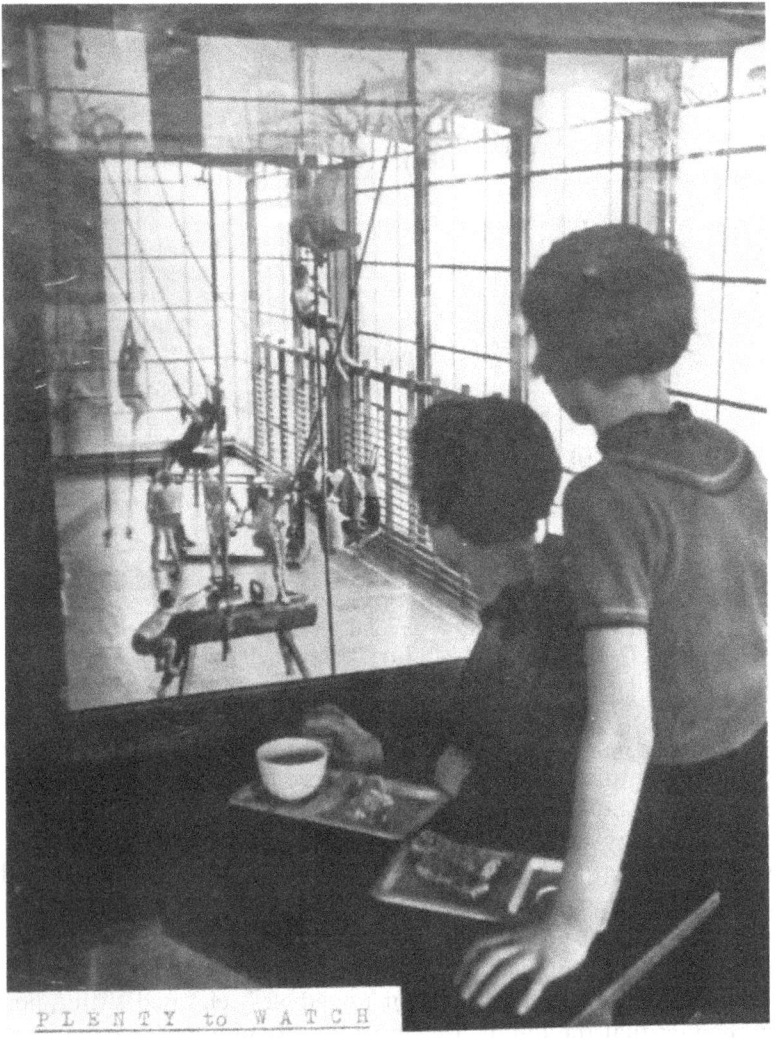

Figure 7.5 "Plenty to watch"
(Innes H. Pearse and Lucy H. Crocker, *The Peckham Experiment. A Study of the* Living *Structure of Society*. London: Allen & Unwin, 1943, 61)

portrayed in a state of nature of sorts. They are in the process of "digesting" the centre and the knowledge within it.

Moving images: *The Centre*

It is not possible to find out anything about the creators of most of the photographs. We can say more, however, about the genesis of a film that constitutes one of the most fascinating sources on the PHC, namely *The Centre*, a

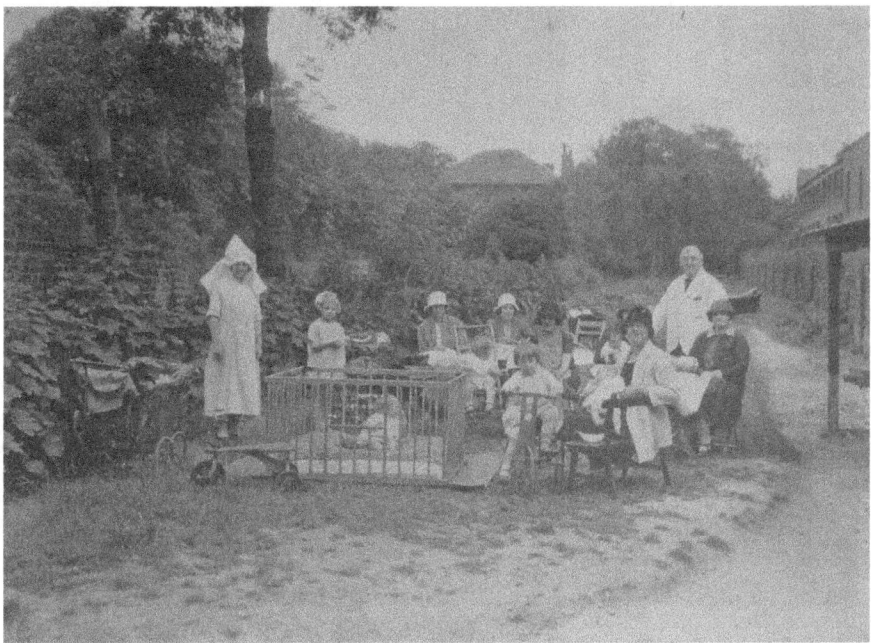

Figure 7.6 In the garden on Queen's Road
(Annual Report 1926, WL, SA/PHC/A.2/1)

1947 documentary on the experiment of just over 20 minutes.[4] It begins with a title sequence superimposed on a map of London, reminiscent, maybe not by chance, of Charles Booth's poverty maps. A male narrator then issues an invitation to travel from the "centre" of London (we see the Parliament buildings on the banks of the Thames) to the "centre". A whip pan follows several buses and trams heading south over Westminster Bridge in the direction of Peckham. The viewer is given a description of the district and its social milieu, made up mostly of skilled labourers. There are brief glimpses of summery streets: the area seems neat and tidy. The camera finally comes to rest on the PHC building. We then see a number of interior views of the centre, which the narrator characterizes as a unique research project on "human biology" – though he does not explain what this implies. Instead, we are presented with a number of leisure activities available at the centre and are told:

> People don't kill time in the Centre, they use time. They acquire physical and mental health. They can do what they like, when they like, as they like. And in this way the Centre becomes a community of families and not just a mass of individuals.[5]

This first, rather mundane section is followed by a narrative that soon turns out to be a case study explicating the centre's modus operandi. A female

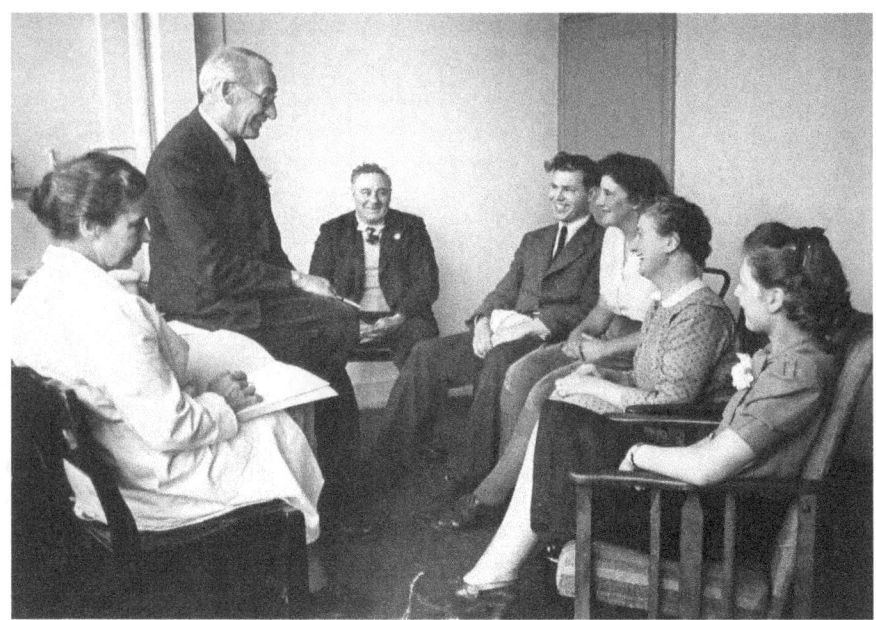

Figure 7.7 A family consultation in the late 1940s
(Health overhaul c. 1920s–1930s, WL, SA/PHC/H.1/4)

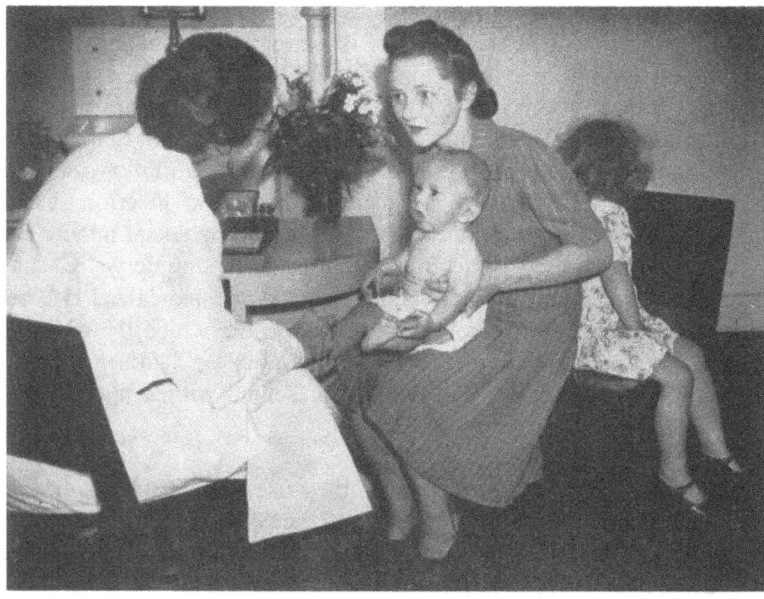

Figure 7.8 "Mother has a question" (1940s)
(Innes H. Pearse, *The Quality of Life: The Peckham Approach to Human Ethology.*
Edinburgh: Scottish Academic Press, 1979, plate 13)

voice-over provides commentary. Both camera and narrator follow the Jones family – Maureen, Fred and their little boy Johnny – from their first visit to the centre to the birth of their second child about a year later. We accompany them during their evening stroll through the brightly lit building and observe them as they in turn observe the peaceful yet bustling life at the centre. They find themselves attracted by gender- and age-specific activities. Fred shows an interest in the darts club, Maureen in the nursery, little Johnny in the games being played by children in the gymnasium. The family takes up membership and is examined by Pearse and Scott Williamson – and here we witness a minor drama: Pearse has to inform Maureen that her pregnancy has caused a cyst, though this is easily removable, requiring only a minor operation. Maureen, however, is shocked by the news and now wants nothing more to do with the centre, though she knows Fred and Johnny are enthusiastic about it. Fred, meanwhile patiently continues to pay the membership fee. In a key scene Maureen then appears at home, clearly immersed in thought – as Pearse's earlier remarks on the centre from the voice-over echo through her mind. Maureen's efforts to come to terms with the situation soon conclude: she decides to have the operation, which is arranged in consultation with the doctors. Now the narrative pace picks up. Following the successful operation Maureen throws herself into life at the centre. The family makes friends, and soon – as the viewer notes when other members teach Maureen how to make suitable clothes – a new baby is on the way.

The narrative might have ended there but instead it continues for a few more minutes, providing us with the most interesting part of the film. Here, during the pregnancy, the camera repeatedly shifts away from the Jones family, roaming through the building, capturing community activities of all kinds: a theatre group's rehearsals, a dance night, a reading. At the same time the commentator's authoritative voice falls silent and sentimental music takes over – perhaps an illustration of the Peckham scientists' hard-to-verbalize, holistic insights?

Pearse and Scott Williamson were in fact involved in the film's genesis beyond their on-screen roles. The original idea for a project of this kind was hatched by renowned producer Paul Rotha, who had been commissioned by the Central Office of Information to produce a series of films on the theme "Britain can make it", and had come across the centre in the course of his research.[6] Funded by the Foreign Office, the film was then shot in 1947, on location at the centre on St Mary's Road, which was turned upside down for several weeks. Not only did the film team eat their way through all the food in the cafeteria, but the building's glass interior walls had to be removed in order to ensure smooth camera movements.[7] Apparently, it was Pearse and Scott Williamson who prompted directors J.B. Holmes and Langton Gould-Marks to make the centre itself the real star.[8] For anyone familiar with their texts there is a temptation to put even the smallest of details in the script down to the medical directors' influence. For example, we are told that: "[T]he gym is filled with boys and girls of all ages, enjoying themselves at various activities – all non-organised."[9] The script thus conveys how neatly – at least for the filming – the lack of organization in the centre was organized. A few pages on it also subtly hints at the knowledge gap between doctors and users. When Maureen is informed of her medical problem, causing her to look pensive, there is a shot of Pearse and Scott Williamson: "They exchange rapid and almost imperceptible glances."[10]

It is interesting to note how *The Centre* stages the researchers' first appearance. The viewer initially gets to see Scott Williamson and Lucy Crocker as observers at an elevated vantage point – namely the balcony overlooking the gymnasium. They are looking through the same window through which, in the image discussed above, two children are watching others at play. The two researchers, however, then descend into the centre and take part in the communicative processes unfolding there. Their final appearance in the film is also noteworthy. We see Scott Williamson, this time with Pearse, not in his lab coat or evaluating data at his desk but in casual attire. The medical directors are bidding farewell to a family and are clearly in the act of mixing with centre users. We discover nothing specific about how research was carried out at the centre. One scene showing tickets being handed out was cut.[11]

The directors of the film met with members as well in order to recruit extras but also in an attempt to make the film more realistic through their input. This is a remarkable procedure: a film team contacts the participants in a social experiment to ask their advice on how to most authentically portray their own spontaneous behaviour. The minutes of their meeting, however, reveal an instructive conflict between members that shows how differently they interpreted the experiment. One user suggested starting the film with little Johnny in the street, playing in the dirt. This provoked the ire of another (female) user: this was make-believe; there had never been anything like that in Peckham.[12] While member *a* was keen to introduce a classical motif of social work – the slum child – in order to convey the centre's positive impact, member *b* demonstrated a loyalty to her neighbourhood, while also showing a class pride to which the centre directors' texts and the film itself attached little importance.

A winter evening

The pictures from Peckham are staged, even the snapshots. We can get a sense of this, finally, from an impressionistic examination of a photograph in *The Quality of Life*. It is captioned "The Cafeteria: early on a winter evening" and appears to show a relaxed, everyday scene at the centre (Figure 7.9). We see a pleasant jumble of furnishings and different types of people; the photo comes across as a random sample of real life at the centre, as also implied by the non-specific title.

Then, however, to the lower right of the image we notice the photographer's silhouette and the dark shadow cast on the column at the back by a woman carrying a child. We grasp how bright the light illuminating them must have

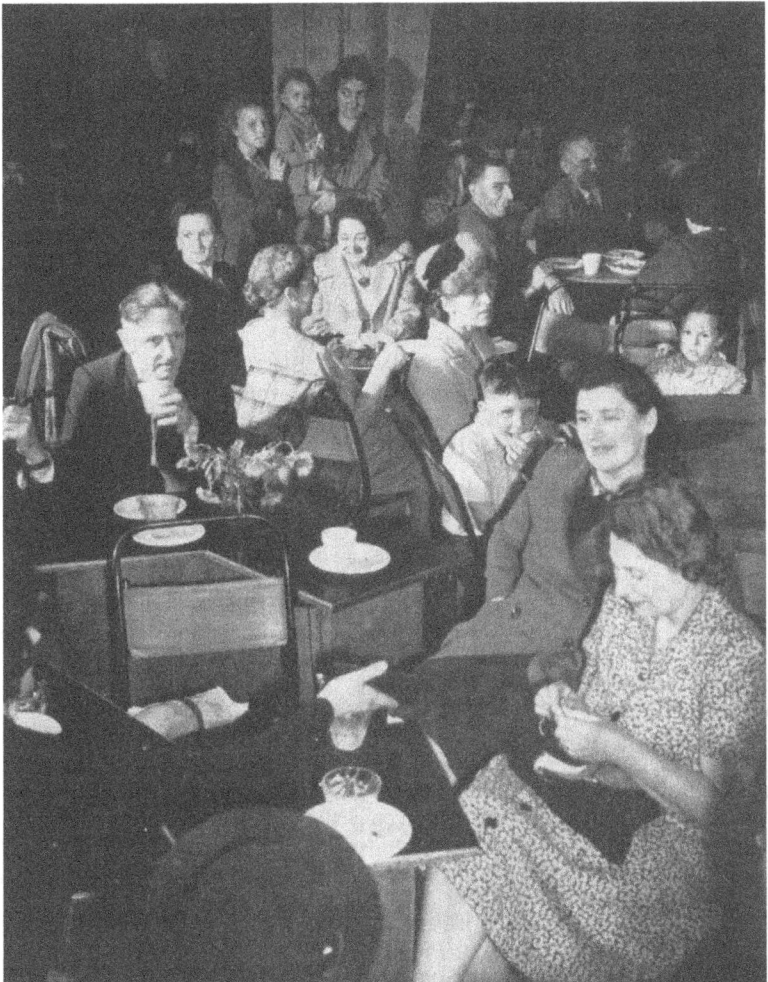

Figure 7.9 The photographer's shadow
(Innes H. Pearse, *The Quality of Life: The Peckham Approach to Human Ethology.*
Edinburgh: Scottish Academic Press, 1979, plate 9)

been. And suddenly it becomes clear that the adults shown here were
captured while engaged in everyday activities, conversing with each other,
sipping from a cup or sewing. In other words they appear to be taking no
notice whatsoever of the photographer. All the children in the picture, however, are looking directly at him, betraying his own influence on the scene –
and involuntarily revealing that most of the individuals shown knew precisely
how they were supposed to conduct themselves. We are dealing with a situation saturated by interpretations of what was happening at the Pioneer Health
Centre on the part of all those involved. In the Peckham Experiment – as we

will see in the next chapter – a subtle form of intervention by scientists in the lives of ordinary people came up against their complex pertinacity as they sought to come to terms with this very encounter.

Notes

1 See above all: Photos, SLHA, PC 613, and WL, SA/PHC/H.1.
2 In the late 1940s Pearse and Scott Williamson contemplated making use of photographs to analyse users' choice of partner with regard to physical attributes and social status, aligning the findings with those of hormonal examinations. This is one of the few pieces of evidence that they considered how one might keep instincts and social influences separate. They did not implement this plan: Research programme. October 1949, WL, SA/PHC/B.5/10.
3 Pearse and Crocker, *The Peckham Experiment*, 51–66.
4 Online at: "The Centre", https://player.bfi.org.uk/free/film/watch-the-centre-1947-on line (accessed December 17, 2017).
5 *The Centre*, 2'25"–2'42".
6 Minutes of the Meeting held at Pioneer Health Centre – Peckham to discuss the proposed Film about the Centre, undated [1946], WL, SA/PHC/B.5/18/1, 2.
7 Donaldson to Winfrey, June 21, 1947, WL, SA/PHC/B.5/15.
8 Minutes of the Meeting held at Pioneer Health Centre – Peckham to discuss the proposed Film about the Centre, WL, SA/PHC/B.5/18/1, 3. Initially, the film-makers had planned to kick off with a moderator in a studio who would then visit the centre and speak with those in charge. Different users, they envisaged, would then present specific spaces: Treatment by Langton Gould-Marks, May 3, 1946, WL, SA/PHC/B.5/.
9 Notes for Draft Shooting Script Part Three, May 28, 1947, WL, SA/PHC/B.5/18/1, 6.
10 Ibid., 21. The Jones family itself was a blend of reality and fiction. The actors were laypeople and members of the centre. "Fred", played by fireman Fred Scarsie, was in fact Johnny's father, but "Maureen", the teacher Olga Smith, was not his mother – the filmmakers thought her too tall for the role. Here "biology" was clearly less important than aesthetics: leaflet on the premiere, undated [1947], WL, SA/PHC/B.5/18/1.
11 Notes for Draft Shooting Script Part Three, May 28, 1947, WL, SA/PHC/B.5/18/1.
12 Minutes of the Meeting held at Pioneer Health Centre – Peckham to discuss the proposed Film about the Centre, undated [c. 1946], WL, SA/PHC/B.5/18/1, 10.

8 Guinea pigs?

The members between participation and social control

Long before the filming of *The Centre*, radio had discovered the Peckham Experiment.[1] In 1937 Howard Marshall, a popular sports broadcaster (and later expert on personnel management) reported on the PHC within the framework of a BBC series dedicated to social experiments. Marshall asked surprisingly critical questions about the centre, which, as it happens, reminded him of a ship. He interviewed Scott Williamson in the consulting room: "The doctors here will tell you that it's the first biological research station in the world – actually it's a family club."[2] Scott Williamson agreed: the main purpose of the project was the observation of entirely normal people. Marshall pressed him: "Do you mean that this great building is a sort of bait to tempt your material inside?" Though Scott Williamson had admitted just that on more than one occasion, he denied that it was. Marshall also asked whether families' exclusive access to the centre was not unfair towards single people. Scott Williamson, passing over the objectives of the first centre, responded: "Perhaps it is, but we haven't come here to be kind but to conduct a scientific experiment."

Marshall also talked to Lucy Crocker about her approach to the children: "I suppose you have to provide them with opportunity. How do you decide what to offer them?" Crocker: "I don't. You watch them carefully and then follow the hints they give you." The children, she explained, then pursued activities that enriched them physically and psychologically, and this they did in a completely autonomous way. Here Marshall became suspicious: "Well, it all seems rather complicated to me. And a bit contradictory. You talk about the family organism and say you mustn't consider the child separately; and then you talk about each member of the family as an individual." Crocker responded evasively: "It's very early days yet. But it's an apparent paradox – actually it's all part of the growth of a complex organism." Marshall was not entirely convinced: "I'm not sure [...] how much this Centre depends upon the personality of the doctors who started it and who are carrying it on now." He concluded with a tricky question to his listeners: "Do you agree that it's important that people should be responsible for their own health by joining a Centre of this kind and paying a subscription? Or do you think work of this kind should be voluntary – charitable, that's to say – or state organised?"[3]

The statements of Scott Williamson and Crocker clearly did nothing to make this question any easier to answer, as evident in a critical review of the broadcast in the *Manchester Guardian*. The reviewer was irritated by the researchers' platitudes. They should, he contended, explain in more detail what exactly they were investigating.[4]

Howard Marshall, however, not only gave the researchers their say but also wanted to hear from the users of the centre. Over a coffee he chatted with Mrs Cunningham, who explained that she had been a member for one month and would like to get all her acquaintances to come along: "I think the finest thing about it is that there isn't any class distinction. I like seeing the doctors line up to get their food at the cafeteria like everybody else."[5] Mrs Wilson had been there for a year, felt much healthier already and recapitulated: "Coming here sort of freed me, you know. Why, I don't know myself." Finally, Mr Newman was also fascinated by the research project itself: "[I] can see there's a far greater thing behind it. [...] I'm gradually getting to understand what it's all about." Marshall wondered: "You don't mind being part of an experiment?" Newman: "No, it's very interesting. [...] I've never had the chance of making contact with people like the doctors here."[6] From the perspective of the members Marshall spoke to, then, the centre was a complete success. By 1937 they were already referring to increased social integration and health, observing the experiment's effects on themselves. This is no surprise: after all, at the time of the broadcast it was quite possible for centre members to be well acquainted with the experiment's progress, especially if they attended the Sunday meetings at which Scott Williamson urged them to study themselves.

Members' memoirs

The search for other responses to this call for study of the self brings us to interviews carried out in the 1980s. This was the high point of former centre staff's above-mentioned efforts to transform the "kaleidoscope of events" there into "meaningful concepts", to quote the minutes of one meeting.[7] In 1984 journalist John Nye was tasked with collating former users' recollections. These are unlikely to have been of much help to the former staff members. Nye summarized the results as follows: the people enjoyed reminiscing about the centre, but they had barely understood the research carried out there. What they recalled in the main was the project's service aspect, for example, how efficiently people were referred to hospitals in case of illness. There was little here to substantiate grand biological theories, and the same goes for statements by members such as "it was all very well organized" and "[w]e appreciated it because we couldn't afford anything else".[8] Above all, however, these recollections make it clear who had the final say within the centre. One user even recalled: "My husband was told off terribly because he hit this boy."[9]

Five years later, Alison Stallibrass, former assistant to Crocker, published a book on the centre. In the main it paraphrases *The Peckham Experiment*, its key goal – as already evident in the title, *Being Me and Also Us* – the corroboration of the claim that self-realization is always conducive to social integration. What makes the book interesting is that it seeks to prove what Stallibrass considers to be the most important of the "Lessons from the Peckham Experiment" (to quote the subtitle), with the help of two chapters containing "Members' Memoirs". Stallibrass interviewed a number of ex-users between 1978 and 1985. As if to demonstrate the centre's long-term effects, their statements were preceded by biographical sketches. Without exception, these are success stories of social advancement, engagement in civil society and happy marriages. Ethelyn Hazell, for example, had founded an organic agribusiness in the 1970s and had written a book about it. Wally Arnold had joined a group whose members built their own houses without professional help.[10]

In contrast to Nye's interviews most of these memoirs are wholly positive about the centre. Many are in fact moving. Often they describe a happy phase in people's lives featuring intensive friendships. Even in Stallibrass's heavily edited collection of quotations, however, we get a sense that members had differing views on the freedoms at the centre. For example, Rose Runcers supplemented her friend Lily Mears's enthusiastic remark that "[the Centre] was run by the people" by stating: "I do feel we did want a bit more discipline. Especially the children." It is also noteworthy that almost all Stallibrass's interviewees had been in fairly close contact with the centre's staff. Adge Elven, for example, was involved in the distribution of the tickets; Hazell typed for Mary Langman; Elsie Purser helped guide groups of visitors through the centre. This makes their accounts of their own development all the more fascinating, if less representative of the average member's experience. John Smith mentions that as a young boy he had learned a great deal at the centre simply by watching others, which had fostered his "personality development". Gladys Coring made very similar statements – "The Centre gave you confidence"– as did Sally Woodhouse: "We all sort of grew and expanded in ways you would never have thought of." Mears recalled: "You got a sense of being your own self. You got the habit of thinking 'I could do that'. You got the power to take responsibility. I am sure I have done much more with my life." And May Burnett remarked: "[It] provided opportunities for us all; [...] no-one made you do anything, but if you saw something and it suddenly stirred you to some kind of action ..."[11]

In light of these statements it seems as if the centre's influence on these individuals, at least over the long term, consisted in encouraging them to reflect on their own development – and in doing so to use certain terms popular among the researchers, such as "pattern", "responsibility", and "potential". It is, of course, difficult to determine whether they had already picked up this terminology in the 1940s, when Pearse and Scott Williamson allowed it to percolate into the centre, whether these terms had simply become common by the early 1980s or whether former users deployed them because they had read books on the centre. In any event, Elven's 1989 remarks on the users' children do seem like something borrowed from the *The Peckham Experiment*:

[L]eaping about, swinging on the ropes and devising our own games [...] [, w]e used the apparatus generally as it should not be used. We just played. [...] The children had the freedom to choose. It was interesting to see the pattern of activity of the children – when they joined, rushing about and trying everything and then settling into an individual pattern.[12]

It is also interesting to note how he sums up his recollections: "[The children] were all searching all the time for what they wanted."[13] Once again this sounds highly up to date: for Elven, Peckham helped people explore their own wants and interests.

Borrowings from the Peckham researchers' thinking and vocabulary are most apparent in Stallibrass's interview with Elsie Purser. Her parents were among the first residents of Peckham to become members of the centre in 1935. Purser recalls having been bored and lonely before that. At the centre she then became "a personality, not just a number or another patient; I was ME". After the war she began to take a strong interest in the experiment. She also attended Scott Williamson's talks, which she portrays in a highly emotional, almost religious language. In her account the very moments when Scott Williamson sought to turn centre members into his scientific colleagues were aglow with love, indescribable. Nonetheless, Purser's raptures were probably intended to back up the book's interpretation of the centre. She knew exactly what was expected of her as an interviewee. While her fellow ex-member Gladys Coring expressed the view that the experiment had been unique, in part due to the directors' personalities, Purser was firmly convinced that such a centre could also be established elsewhere and with different personnel.[14]

It is not my intention to question the genuine enthusiasm felt by the people Stallibrass talked to. But anyone who spends some time studying "Peckham" will note that it is always the same interviewees who crop up in the documents. Right up to the present Adge Elven's wife Pam, for example, has helped disseminate the lessons of the Peckham Experiment as secretary of the aforementioned Pioneer Health Foundation; and she was even involved in ensuring the survival of records relevant to the centre.[15] Clearly, the contemporary witnesses discussed here constitute a small group of individuals who were already grappling intensively with the experiment while it was underway.[16] Inevitably, then, Stallibrass's oral history is blind to the fact that not all those involved contributed to the research with the same passion for experimentation. In the Wellcome Library, for example, we find a 1936 letter from a Mrs Bridger informing Pearse of her decision to stop coming to the centre. Bridger was unhappy with the way other children were influencing her daughter: "[I]n Betty's case we find that it is always she who is influenced by children in a lower social scale than herself."[17] In her response Pearse ignored the potential for conflict at the centre so openly addressed here – the fact that for users social mixing did not necessarily mean mutual appreciation. Instead she began to pontificate in an almost accusatory tone: "We believe, as you would have heard had you come to your family consultation, – that the main duty of parents is the weaning of the child."[18] In the archive's collection of cuttings we also find a reader's letter, signed by an "ex-member" (and unfortunately undated), on the "failure of the Peckham Health Centre". It too suggests a less harmonious history: because nothing is organized at the centre, new members are left out in the cold unless they already know someone before joining.[19] Finally, the image of anarchical-convivial self-organization on St Mary's Road is tarnished when we learn from the local press that the centre could be a genuine risk to safety. In 1947 a teenager drowned in the unmonitored pool while the curator was distributing tickets.[20] Two years later a four-year-old boy, left in the sole charge of his sister, fell from the first-floor balcony and was in a coma for several days.[21]

"Bouquets & Brickbats"

The most striking source on users' view of the centre are the six issues of the members' magazine *The Guinea Pig* from 1948, along with its successor *The Centre* (Figure 8.1), which appeared in late 1949 and early 1950.[22] The name itself is grandiose: what kind of guinea pigs produce a magazine about themselves? The kind who enjoy being studied, as it turns out. Comparison of the individuals involved in Stallibrass's book and the magazine, which was published more than 40 years earlier, is instructive. The editors and main authors were none other than Norbert ("Nobby") Clarke, Ron Goldsmith – and Elsie Purser.

The Guinea Pig was a fairly professional production. For three pence readers got a dozen pages, consisting mostly of columns informing them about events at the centre. Organizational matters received attention in the shape, for example, of monthly programmes and personal ads for dancing partners. Members were congratulated on their success in tennis or boxing or on getting married and there were detailed reports on the film about the centre and those appearing in it. Above all, the magazine was pervaded with allusions to individuals' lovable quirks, mildly salacious gags and friendly taunts between the clubs.[23] The swing club, for example, challenged the classical music fans to a debate.[24] The members of the swimming club gleefully reported their victory over the darts club at darts; the latter responded that while it was true that they had been narrowly beaten, they had achieved a draw against the table tennis club, which they were now thinking of challenging to a table tennis match.[25] With reference to the football club Purser and Goldsmith wrote: "If you want to contact them, find a group that looks like a debating society; that should be them."[26] The tone was generally friendly and humorous; but even the jokes express the Peckham norm: the positive affirmation of amateurism, of trying things out.[27]

The Guinea Pig, however, also makes it clear that being a mere member of the Pioneer Health Centre did not automatically make one a diligent participant in the Peckham Experiment. The magazine pulled no punches in addressing those

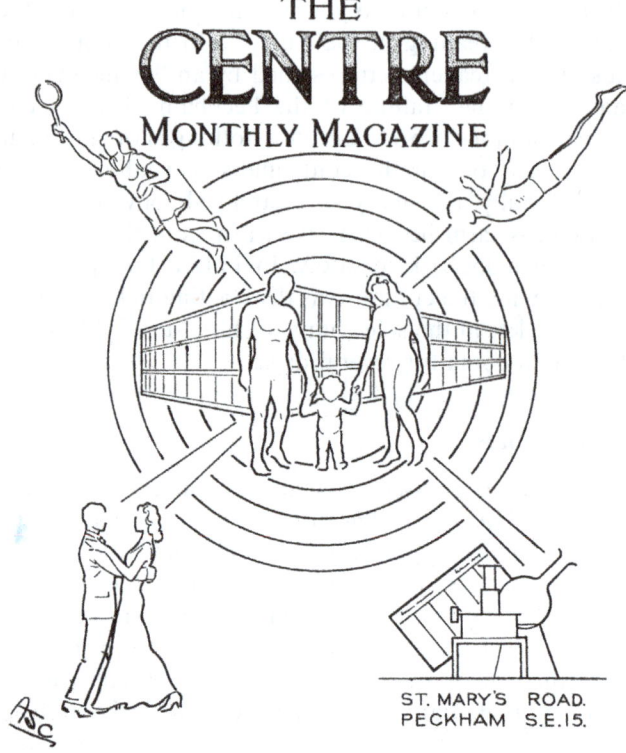

Figure 8.1 The graphic alignment of nuclear family and health centre
(*The Centre Monthly Magazine* (September 1949), WL, SA/PHC/B.5/12, cover image)

who had been coming to the centre only since its post-war reopening, implicitly accusing them of having failed to understand its scientific objectives.[28] Time and again contributors lamented the loss of the "centre spirit" that had prevailed during its first years.[29] Clearly, *The Guinea Pig* intended to help build a centre identity. But it was also a monthly call to order. This is especially evident in a column entitled "Bouquets & Brickbats", which also reveals that even the post-war centre was plagued by a degree of disorderly conduct. Warnings were issued, for example, to individuals who hammered on toilet doors, used hoses for swinging or failed to return dishes to their proper place.[30] Apparently, in 1948 a gang of youths wearing brown trilby hats made members feel unsafe for a time.[31] Teenage members were informed of Scott Williamson's concerns that more and more outsiders were being allowed into the centre. It was not a "dance hall": "The adolescents must learn to use it as their club."[32] Here we discern the limits to freedom at the centre. Its central premise was non-negotiable: only families were allowed in. Yet it was users themselves who enforced this rule. The magazine editors, meanwhile, bemoaned – one of their brickbats – the paltry number of individuals turning up at Scott Williamson's talks.[33]

Rather than shoring up its external borders, the "Icebreakers" column was devoted to overcoming barriers within the centre. Drawing on metaphors of warmth and closeness, it encouraged members to push through interpersonal obstacles ("Break the Ice and be friendly"). Allusions were made to one lovestruck member who, it was suggested, should finally pluck up the courage to talk to the object of his affection. From the fifth issue, however, the column was accompanied by a striking illustration, which demonstrates that it was possible to interpret the imperative for integration in far more martial fashion (Figure 8.2): rather than an invitation to communicate, here the icebreaker was visualized as a man scattering a clique with a stick. In fact, on a number of occasions *The Guinea Pig* presses users to refrain from establishing exclusive social circles. The members of a badminton group, for example, were given a ticking-off for sequestering themselves behind a closed door. They were even encouraged to comment on the issue in the magazine.[34]

Evidently, there was a code of conduct at the Pioneer Health Centre that at least some members adhered to and tried to impart to others. It seems likely that the centre's staff looked favourably on members who behaved like good experimental participants, in other words those who were active, welcomed interaction with other people and who had an enquiring, open-minded attitude to their own development. What the researchers observed at the centre, then,

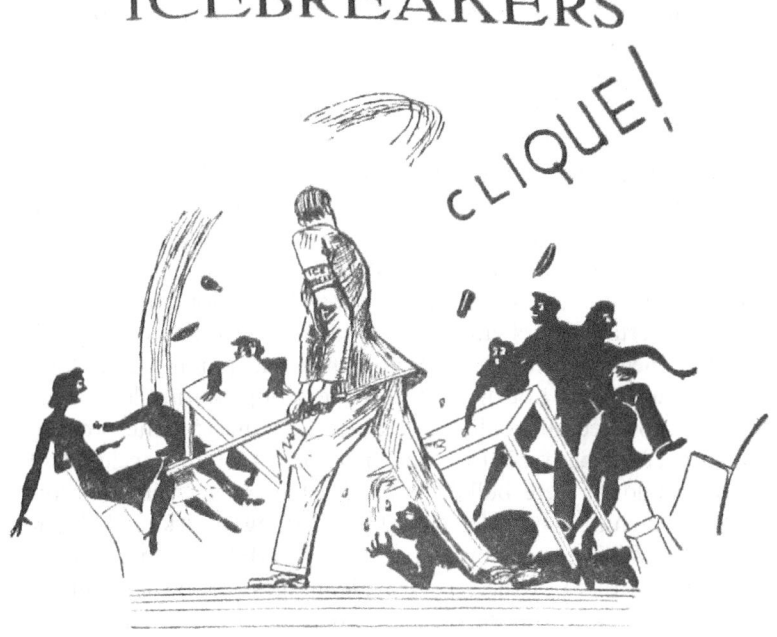

Figure 8.2 The "Icebreaker" at work. Note the official-looking armband (*The Guinea Pig* 5 (1948), WL, SA/PHC/B.5/12, 11)

was by no means natural, even going by their own interpretation of the term. It was the effect of complex, sometimes conflict-laden dynamics that arose when their interpretations came up against the individual expectations and interests of the members, some of whom made these interpretations their own.[35]

An experiment in education

It should be clear by now that the children involved in the Peckham Experiment were subject to particularly close observation. As the directors saw it, they represented raw biological potential, uninfluenced by alienating civilization. By studying them they hoped to be able to investigate, from a long-term perspective, the expansion of their spheres of interest and realms of action – a process with its own inherent logic, marked by specific periods of "appetite" – while also observing the resulting increase in their vitality. Time and again the books of Pearse and Scott Williamson tell of children free of fear, mixing well even with adults and quite capable of drawing on life at the centre as they saw fit.[36] In contrast, the institution of the school stood for standardized learning forced upon isolated age-based groups – even a kind of force-feeding detrimental to health. Like the policeman, the traditional teacher had become the epitome of all those unnatural structures it was so crucial to combat.[37] It thus comes as no surprise that by the 1930s the directors had encountered the ideas of Maria Montessori. In 1938 Scott Williamson gave members of the London Montessori Society a tour through the building, which they were evidently delighted with.[38] The annual report of 1938–1939 mentioned that a joint educational experiment had been agreed upon – the centre would provide the rooms and Montessori the teachers' salaries. This collaboration, however, was scuppered by the outbreak of war.[39]

When the centre reopened its directors returned to the idea of a school, in part, apparently, on the initiative of a number of parents. The so-called Centre School only existed for a short time, and just a few members sent their children there.[40] However, it serves as another powerful example of the limits to the project's freedom: it is in the sources on the school that we find the only evidence that certain users attempted to co-govern the centre – without success. At a meeting with Scott Williamson the parents complained that their children, who were not divided into age groups during lessons and were provided with no fixed curriculum, were not learning to write properly. They were also concerned because there had been several minor accidents. Finally, the youngest children were bullied by their older peers, who – according to the directors' teachings – should have been serving as a knowledge resource for them. Scott Williamson, however, failed to address the parents' concerns, instead reminding them of the school's advantages – elsewhere children were forced to sit still – and assuring them that they need only wait for the desired results to occur: "If the parents are continually wanting something from other worlds it can't be done."[41] Nonetheless, the parents demanded the right to bring in someone from outside with proper teacher training. This was out of the question for Scott Williamson. Such an individual would first have to unlearn their training: "I have the same difficulty in training my staff in the medical department (so that they do not work as ordinary doctors)." He concluded with an authoritative declaration: "Your children may not be backward in the power for living, though they may be backward in the A.B.C."[42]

Notes

1 The BBC followed the centre's progress over the course of its existence. In the late 1940s its offshoots carried reports on "Peckham" to every corner of the Commonwealth: see various scripts in: WL, SA/PHC/B.5/17/2.
2 It's Happening Now: The Pioneer Health Centre, Peckham: Howard Marshall and others; draft and script, January 4, 1937, WL, SA/PHC/B.3/18, 4.
3 Quotations: ibid., 4–5, 9–10, 21–22.
4 "Review of Broadcasting", *The Manchester Guardian* (June 1, 1937).
5 It's Happening Now: The Pioneer Health Centre, Peckham: Howard Marshall and others; draft and script, January 4, 1937, WL, SA/PHC/B.3/18, 13.
6 Ibid., 15, 17.
7 Minutes, Health Committee, February 19, 1980, WL, SA/PHC/C.14/2.
8 Reminiscences of St Mary's Road Peckham, June/October 1984, WL, SA/PHC/C.20, Appendix 1.
9 Ibid., Appendix 4.
10 Stallibrass, *Being Me and Also Us*, 138, 144.
11 Ibid., quotations: 141, 123, 124–125, 149, 145, 134.
12 Ibid., 128–129.
13 Ibid. One statement in Nye's interviews is also consonant with Elven's assessment. Gladys Coring mentions that Scott Williamson often questioned users about why they had not tried out a particular activity until they stated clearly that they did not *want* to: Reminiscences of St Mary's Road Peckham, June/October 1984, WL, SA/PHC/C.20, 6.
14 Stallibrass, *Being Me and also Us*, 152, 58, 146, 158.
15 Hall, *The Archives of the Pioneer Health Centre*. See Pam Elven, Written testimony, "It Seems Only Yesterday", September 3, 2009, and "Unique Experience 1935–1950", undated, SLHA, PC 613. Elven also contributed to the BBC documentary *Health before the NHS: The Road to Recovery* (2016), mentioned in the introduction – which, as it happens, made use of excerpts from *The Centre* without further comment.
16 What we encounter here are the typical methodological problems involved in portraying medical relationships "from below". See: Anne Borsay and Peter Shapley, eds, *Medicine, Charity and Mutual Aid. The Consumption of Health and Welfare in Britain, c. 1550–1950* (Aldershot: Ashgate, 2007).
17 Bridger to Pearse, June 10, 1936, WL, SA/PHC/B.3/7/7–8.
18 At play here, Pearse concluded, is an environment in which the child himself is confronted with decisions that the adults eventually have to let him make alone. Pearse to Bridger, June 20, 1936, WL, SA/PHC/B.3/7/7–8.
19 Cuttings books, 1938–1941, WL, SA/PHC/A.3/3.
20 "Boy loses Life at Peckham Health Centre", *London Observer* (June 25, 1947).
21 *South London Advertiser* (August 26, 1949).
22 Unfortunately there are no extant copies of *The Hub*, a magazine published in the 1930s.
23 Even the centre directors were subject to gossip. For example, in 1948 there were rumours about a certain "Caroline", who was thought to be romantically involved with "Doc Willy": *The Guinea Pig* 5 (1948), 11, WL, SA/PHC/B.5/12/1.

24 *The Guinea Pig* 2 (1948), 3, WL, SA/PHC/B.5/12/1.
25 *The Guinea Pig* 3 (1948), 10, WL, SA/PHC/B.5/12/1.
26 *The Guinea Pig* 6 (1948), 3, WL, SA/PHC/B.5/12/1.
27 *The Guinea Pig* 1 (1948), without page number, WL, SA/PHC/B.5/12/1. The researchers and staff members had their own column, headed "Lab-Oratory", probably an ironic comment on Scott Williamson's missionary style (he wrote the first piece).
28 See esp. the editorial in *The Guinea Pig* 1 (1948), without page number, WL, SA/PHC/B.5/12/1.
29 *The Guinea Pig* 5 (1948), 1, WL, SA/PHC/B.5/12/1.
30 *The Guinea Pig* 1 (1948), 8, WL, SA/PHC/B.5/12/1.
31 Ibid.
32 *The Guinea Pig* 7 (1948), 3, WL, SA/PHC/B.5/12/1.
33 *The Guinea Pig* 1 (1948), 8, WL, SA/PHC/B.5/12/1.
34 *The Guinea Pig* 3 (1948), 3, WL, SA/PHC/B.5/12/1.
35 Such conflicts intensified shortly before the end of the experiment. In 1950, in an article by member J.W. Smith in the *South London Observer*, another unnamed member was chided as selfish. The individual involved had welcomed the idea of opening the centre up to outsiders, which would have ensured its survival, but which Pearse and Scott Williamson saw as incompatible with their research project (see Chapter 10). Smith was certain that he was referring to the majority of users when he wrote: "[T]hey realise that the time and energy expended in establishing the Pioneer Health Centre at Peckham was not in order to make it possible for Mr. and Mrs. 'X' to play billiards and tennis twice a week […] but to study health and development of families living in a special society embracing people of all religious, political views and incomes": J.W. Smith, "Selfish Approach", *South London Observer* (March 10, 1950).
36 Pearse and Crocker, *The Peckham Experiment*, 185.
37 Innes Pearse, Autarchy at Peckham, 1951, WL, SA/PHC/D.2/20.
38 GSW to members of the Montessori Society during visit, October 31, 1938, WL, SA/PHC/D.2/4/4; "A visit to the Pioneer Health Centre", *Montessori Society Quarterly* (October 31, 1938): 2. *The Peckham Experiment* also received rave reviews in: *The Montessori News Bulletin* (September 7, 1944).
39 Annual Reports, 1938/39, WL, SA/PHC/A.2/11, 13.
40 *The Guinea Pig* makes reference to 32 children: *The Guinea Pig* 5 (1948), WL, SA/PHC/B.5/12. The school is one of the aspects of the centre that has been described in a fair amount of detail: Charkin, *"He swings where there is space"*.
41 School – parents' meeting with GSW, January 8, 1948, WL, SA/PHC/B.5/6, 3.
42 Ibid., 4, 7. The documents on the centre's school also contain one of the few indications that Scott Williamson compared his own project with others. In passing, he referred to A.S. Neill's Summerhill reform school, which was founded in 1921 and administered by the pupils, when he complained that his situation was akin to that of Neill: "[H]e only gets the peculiar children of peculiar people." Ibid., 4.

9 Missed opportunities
The centre and the welfare state (1939–1946)

During the Second World War a debate took off in the United Kingdom on post-war society, centred on the relationship between the welfare state, planning, participation and democracy. The Peckham directors believed this opened up major opportunities to apply their insights. At the same time, in the post-1939 writing period their narrative of centre life in the preceding years, which foregrounded the amazing events that had allegedly occurred there, became firmly established. So it is with the war years that the second, shorter part of this book must begin. I now resume the earlier chronology, continuing to narrate events at the Pioneer Health Centre as well as its institutional history, including the period after its reopening in 1946. Henceforth, however, I devote more attention to its contemporary resonance and long-term impact. Over the course of the 1940s the character of the Peckham Experiment changed once again as it became a transnational media phenomenon.

War, agriculture and family

In 1939 the project's media impact could scarcely have been foreseen. The annual report painted a gloomy picture for the first time. It had, it explained, proved necessary to close the centre because it was too costly to black it out and it lacked an air raid shelter. There had also been scientific problems. Many families had been torn apart when the men were called up, ruining the experiment's statistical basis.[1] In fact the centre was subject to a regulation prohibiting large numbers of people from congregating in any buildings that might represent a security risk in the event of an aerial attack on London. This was clearly the case due to the many glass elements in the building's design, and particularly because it was near potential targets in the industrial areas south-east of the Thames. The *Medical Officer* journal stated in 1940: "It is grimly fitting that the Peckham centre should be the first casualty of the Nazi war for it represented an ideal of British Democracy – the care of the family by the family for the family."[2] In accordance with the Emergency Powers Defence Act, the building came under the control of the armed forces and was soon rented to the firm Heating Installations Ltd., which produced radar and radio equipment for the Royal Air Force (RAF).[3] Apparently no one expected the centre to reopen any time soon: the laboratory materials were donated to the Red Cross, the steel chairs to the National Gallery Concerts and the aluminium crockery to the Ministry of Aircraft Production.[4]

Some years earlier, in 1936, Pearse had leased a country house out of her own pocket. The so-called Centre Home Farm was located in Bromley Common, Kent, not far from London. Originally intended to facilitate extra leisure activities for centre children such as tent camps, the main role of this outpost, which included a small area of arable land, had been as a source of fresh vegetables and unpasteurized milk for the centre kitchen. Pearse and Scott Williamson's nutritional ideology also had a concrete physiological aspect: they were among the pioneers of organic agriculture in the United Kingdom. They had links with the Living Soil Society founded by Lady Evelyn Balfour, who had dedicated herself to the struggle against artificial fertilizer and soil erosion. And they were co-founders of the Soil Association, a body that regarded the provision of healthy food as a national duty – one propagated by Balfour with one eye on post-war planning.[5] There was, however, a critique of civilization at play here as well, specifically a concern for the housewife heating up tinned food, alienated from her true calling.[6]

In September 1939 Lucy Crocker moved to Kent along with around 20 centre mothers and their children, and soon the farm too was being presented as a pilot project of major social importance. Pearse began to develop an "Emergency Evacuation Plan", in which she proposed evacuating women and children to the countryside in view of the looming aerial attacks rather than putting them up in strangers' homes.[7] By 1940 this had morphed into a leaflet entitled "War and the Family" (Figure 9.1), which asserted that it was possible to retain the "vitality of the nation" even in wartime by giving urban women the chance to work on the land.[8] The idea was that this could improve the supply situation for the population as a whole while also preventing women from becoming physically and psychologically stunted. Furthermore, the leaflet contended, this plan could function self-sufficiently, at no cost to society. The leaflet met with a positive response, in the *British Medical Journal* for example.[9] But government agencies were less enthusiastic: Pearse tried in vain to gain official recognition for the farm as a so-called Nursery Centre within the framework of the government's programme for evacuated children.[10] The mothers had already left the house by the end of 1940. In 1941 an annex to the building was struck by a bomb.[11] According to one source at least, many of the documents relating to the Peckham Experiment went up in flames along with it.[12]

"Physician, heal thyself"

Around the same time fundamental debates on welfare policy kicked off in the political sphere and press. These debates influenced the famous Beveridge Report, which in turn laid the ground for the massive expansion of the British

War and the Family

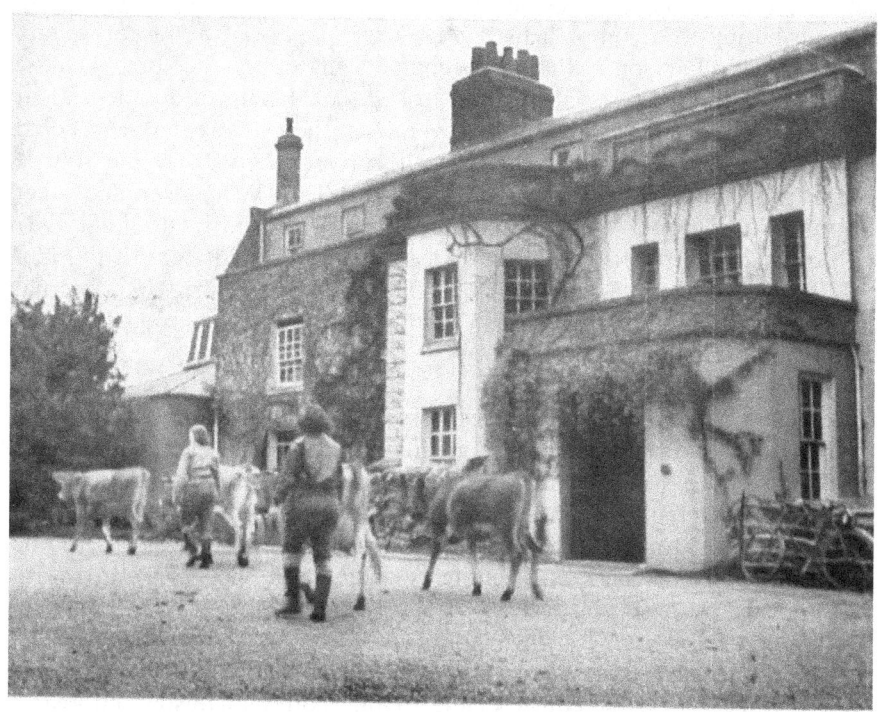

THE CENTRE HOME FARM,

OAKLEY HOUSE,

BROMLEY COMMON, KENT.

May, 1940.

Figure 9.1 The Centre Home Farm
("War and the Family" by Innes Pearse and Lucy Crocker, 1940, WL, SA/PHC/B.4/8/
1, cover image)

welfare state in the post-war period. Health care was one of the main topics
in these debates, which received crucial impulses from Political and Economic
Planning (PEP), a lobbying organization co-founded by Julian Huxley. It is
an interesting indication of the diversity of political ideas from which these
debates drew that Scott Williamson and Pearse in fact contributed to the PEP
Health Group for a short time.[13] As early as 1928 this group had developed
the first plans for a comprehensive health care system. With the appearance
of Scott Williamson and Pearse in 1935, however, a surprising rejection of
state intervention began to creep into the memoranda.[14] Apparently a

number of those involved in the Health Group were soon asking themselves what role such beliefs could possibly play in an organization dedicated to issues of planning and administration.[15] The following year, when the group was contributing to a comprehensive PEP draft paper on the future welfare system, Scott Williamson – who had become its chairman – deplored what he perceived as its rampant socialism and extolled the advantages of independent welfare facilities.[16] He was absent, however, from the meeting that considered the division of responsibilities between the private sector and the state.[17] A major rift appears to have opened up between Scott Williamson and other members of the group. While "Peckham" was mentioned in the final 1937 PEP Report on the British Health Services, a position paper entitled "Planning" from 1944 featured just one brief reference to the centre.[18] An internal memorandum stated that the Health Group had too often become bogged down in debates on principles:

> Dr. Scott Williamson is an idealist possessed of a missionary spirit, while the inquiry and the Report were greatly assisted by his clear conceptions of the needs of a reorientated health service, he was not a suitable person to guide a factual and important inquiry over the whole range of these services. [...] Moreover, the Peckham staff were only concerned with one or two problems and as scientific workers were not concerned with administrative problems.[19]

Here, for the first time, we see a pattern emerging that was to become ever more pronounced over the course of the 1940s. Scott Williamson and Pearse were asked for their expert opinion due to their practical experience providing welfare services. They left behind irritated interlocutors, however, due to their grand biological theories and the conclusions they came to in light of them – which were increasingly hostile to administration. These conclusions are all the more striking when we consider that state interventionist approaches had become increasingly popular from the mid 1930s on, not least among the Peckham researchers' kindred spirits in the reform eugenics movement (one example being the Population Investigation Committee, which had collaborated with the PEP in 1938).

The PHC directors' dissenting views became especially apparent from 1944 on, when Minister of Health Henry Willink presented a White Paper setting out proposals for a comprehensive, tax-funded approach to health care. This laid the ground for the National Health Service Act and thus, in 1948, for the post-war British health care system.[20] The White Paper took up suggestions publicized by the BMA and the aforementioned Beveridge Report (though, unlike the White Paper, both came out in favour of a contribution-funded social insurance system). Amongst these suggestions was the establishment of health centres. The way in which this was to be done, however, prompted Scott Williamson and his colleagues to protest; they even began to monopolize the term "health centre" for their own project.[21] The White Paper envisaged health centres as small polyclinics or joint practices,[22] which would form the local basis for the national system – making them "ill-health centre polyclinics" in the view of the Peckham medical directors.[23] In February 1944, in a series of articles in the *News Chronicle* entitled "What Experts are Saying about the Health Plan", Scott Williamson also gave his views on Willink's proposals. He picked them to pieces: every aspect of Willink's plans, he contended, was plagued by remnants of the old system.[24] In March he was asked by the *British Medical Journal* to fill out a questionnaire on the White Paper but declined to do so, instead criticizing its premise that a state system of compulsory insurance was inevitable in a reader's letter.[25] In fact, a few weeks earlier – probably as a result of repeated mentions of the Peckham Experiment by its supporter Lord Horder in the House of Lords[26] – Scott Williamson had been asked by the Ministry of Information to provide a brief, 100-word summary of the idea behind his centre, explaining its relevance to a future national health care system. He took the opportunity to set out a vision of a nationwide network of administratively and economically independent health centres and a parallel network of equally autonomous centres for general practitioners.[27]

In his essay *Physician, heal thyself*, published the following year, Scott Williamson then expanded this idea into an alternative to the government's proposals. Here he recommended a voluntary system of social insurance essentially free of the state, which would merely administer the finances. From now on, as he envisaged, clinics too would be managed by lay committees rather than the state.[28] Scott Williamson's vision boiled down to a highly demand-oriented system. Patients would be regarded as their doctors' customers; they would be able to switch doctors at any time and pay for their services directly. Differences in income would be offset by a fund administered by the medical profession itself, to which physicians would pay a compulsory contribution graduated according to their turnover. Scott Williamson regarded these proposals as a "new technique – the government of society by the individual for the individual through the individual".[29]

Generally, and more clearly than in other publications, in this essay Scott Williamson revealed himself to be a liberal, particularly through his choice of an economic metaphor to combat the statism of the government's White Paper. The crucial thing was to avoid "monopolies", which were also central to the plans outlined by new Minister of Health Aneurin Bevan. For Scott Williamson, Bevan was giving institutional form to the belief that order inevitably requires subjugation. This conviction, however, did not prevent Scott Williamson from trying to sell his ideas as socialist – Labour had won the recent election. He touted his proposals variously as a form of "liberal socialism" or "social liberalism", apparently without realizing that, for example, his scepticism about the trades unions (another monopoly), which he clearly expressed in his essay, would hold little appeal for most social democrats. The same applies to his reason for rejecting unemployment insurance. If one fostered the individual talents of future workers, he explained, there would be no unemployment in the first place because everyone would find a job in line with his abilities.

Characteristically, Scott Williamson had nothing to say about the political viability of his plan or the existing legal situation. In any case the greater part of his book was dedicated not to his organizational model but to the Peckham Experiment and a call for doctors to view themselves as "explorer[s] into the unknown" rather than specialists.[30] This also inspired the book's title, which ultimately gave expression to Scott Williamson's belief that the solution to social problems lay not in the political process but in a certain "scientific" attitude towards life.

Neither the BMA – which at least shared Scott Williamson's rejection of state oversight and remuneration of doctors[31] – nor the Ministry of Health, let alone the Socialist Medical Association seriously considered his ideas. The latter in particular is likely to have perceived his proposals as the exact opposite of its own thinking. As it shared much common ground with the LCC Hospital and Medical Services Committee, which was dominated by Labour since its electoral victory of 1934, the SMA had just begun to put its vision into practice in London. The committee certainly embraced social medicine but beyond improved outpatient services it took this to include labour protection laws and housebuilding programmes. It also regarded the efforts being made in London to create a unified and universally accessible health care system as a test case for the nation as a whole. With this in mind it stepped up its criticisms of the voluntary sector – for which Scott Williamson ultimately spoke – which it perceived as redundant, uncoordinated and inefficient.[32]

But the specialist (rather than political) press was also far from enthusiastic about Scott Williamson's book. The reviewer in the *Medical Officer* wrote that Scott Williamson was a radical individualist if not anarchist, contending that his scheme might work in a sect but not in a state.[33] The *British Medical Journal* considered his book out of touch with reality. The *Health Tribune* thundered that Scott Williamson's social liberalism was reactionary nonsense, his hatred of bureaucracy incomprehensible.[34] Probably the harshest thumbs-down came from haematologist L.J. Witts. His appraisal was particularly significant because it made a direct connection between Scott Williamson's essay and his centre, which, according to Witts, had been a failure: "[S]tarting with an excellent idea, the Peckham Workers have unfortunately tried to back it up with loose statements and biological analogies rather than hard facts and dispassionate analyses."[35] Witts went so far as to cite a particularly muddled passage from the essay. Scott Williamson felt compelled to respond, conceding that the passage in question was in "Peckhamese".[36]

Reviews and an enforced reopening

The disappointment must have cut deep: prior to publication Scott William-son had been confident that his book would "raise a political stink and might even stir up the Medical Profession to action".[37] It seems likely that his optimism was rooted in the fact that, two years earlier, *The Peckham Experiment* had been a genuine surprise success. Published in 1943, before the year was out a second edition had appeared; in 1947 a slightly revised seventh edition hit the presses.[38] This popularity was in part the result of intensive marketing. In 1943, in the shape of Mary Gowing, the centre had taken on a full-time public relations officer who extolled the book as a potential source of inspiration for debates in a wide variety of fields.[39] Far more often than Scott Williamson's political essay, *The Peckham Experiment* was in fact embraced as a useful contribution to the debate on the future welfare state, despite its lack, indicated above, of concrete advice for political decision-makers. Various actors used the project's findings to highlight the need for action before going on to explain the advantages of their preferred programme.[40]

Neither Gowing nor the two ex-directors responded to such distorted perspectives as long as they remained positive about the centre. No surprise, then, that before long a number of very different variants of the Peckham story were circulating. For example, *The National Insurance Gazette* under-lined what a good idea the Peckham preventive project was due to its cost efficiency,[41] while the *Church Times* praised the PHC's focus on the family.[42] Meanwhile, medical issues played no role in those texts that drew on the PHC to flesh out their social philosophy – such as a 1944 reader's letter in the Quaker magazine *Peace News*, which claimed that the centre might serve as a corrective in view of the threat to individual liberties posed by the impending "'managerial' or 'planning' state".[43] The scientific press was more reserved about the book than its predecessor *Biologists in Search of Material*, which was even commended in *Nature*[44] – a point I will be returning to in a moment. Nonetheless, *The Peckham Experiment* attracted attention across the entire spectrum from basic research to the periodicals of various professional associations, such as the *Nursing Times, The Lancet* and the aforementioned *Medical Officer*, as well as the journal of the Eugenics Society, the *Eugenics Review*.[45] There is no need to look more deeply into any of these reviews because they either considered only partial aspects of the book or adopted the researchers' ideas without further ado – in some cases, in fact, they were written by the Peckham scientists themselves.[46]

Given this overwhelmingly favourable, at times even euphoric reception of their book, before the war was over Scott Williamson and Pearse believed they would soon be entrusted with major responsibilities. In 1943, for example, they presented a number of their financial backers with a memorandum that envisaged turning the centre into a pure research unit after the war, one that would concurrently train the directors of new centres: a "National Institute for the Study of Health – or the Science of Creative Synthesis", as they called it.[47] The two former directors apparently had much more in mind than simply continuing their work of the late 1930s,[48] despite the urgings of supporters such as Lord Horder and the publisher Stanley Unwin – the latter most likely with his own economic interest in mind.[49]

Ultimately, however, it appears to have been the forces they themselves unleashed that prompted Scott Williamson and Pearse to reopen the old centre. By 1944 a number of ex-members had called a meeting where they discussed how they might ensure its reopening. Mr Hayes, the centre's former doorman, drew up a list of pre-war members and in April 1945 more than 100 of them got together.[50] Immediately after the capitulation of Germany the two directors were invited to a meeting by the former users; a few weeks later the latter issued an appeal to the prime minister to make the unused centre building, which was still under government administration, available. Copies of this petition (in which they also appealed to the government not to squander "British leadership in Social Services and Social Science") were sent to MPs and ministries.[51] Scott Williamson and Pearse themselves appear to have embraced these demands only in August 1945.

The petition was successful and the building was made available for normal use in 1946, with £10,000 from the Halley Stewart Trust, an institution that had previously supported publication of *The Peckham Experiment*, facilitating its reopening.[52] But the centre was in a sorry state. The rooms were contaminated with oil, while most of the furnishings had been given away.[53] Faced with these problems, many former users showed tremendous commitment. Several articles in the local press were accompanied by photographs of cheerful cleaning squads heading into the centre with their pails and brooms. The members also carried out the necessary carpentry work. A party to celebrate the opening was then held on 23 March 1946. While the mayor of Camberwell and supporters such as Lord Geddes and Ewen Montagu gave speeches to mark the occasion,[54] this celebration was clearly very different from the inauguration ceremony a decade earlier: this was a members' party rather than an event for financial backers and dignitaries.[55]

Visitors and lecture tours

The tumultuous events, as Mary Langman called them,[56] that led to the reopening of the centre, reveal the Peckham actors' varied range of motives. For many of its users the centre was a fairly affordable source of medical care and a much-loved recreational facility. For Pearse and Scott Williamson it was a research project and as such, from their perspective, it had already had its day before the war. At the very least we are left with the strong impression that they used the reopened centre chiefly as a walk-in version of their books. From 1946 on it was almost overwhelmed by the mass of visitors,[57] but this does not appear to have prompted the directors to take remedial action. In fact, a meticulously compiled list for the period May to October 1949 records visitors every day. They came from all over the world: Chicago, Oslo, Johannesburg and Berlin, the Netherlands, Finland, Denmark, India, Belgium, Canada, France and Australia. They included teachers, doctors, social workers, delegations sent by political parties, students of sociology and architecture, nurses and journalists.[58] A memorandum from 1947 mentions that the centre had been visited by 4,000 interested parties from 31 countries in the previous 12 months alone, including representatives of UNESCO, the surgeon general of the United States and the deputy health minister of India.[59] Little wonder, then, that this flood of visitors itself became a topic of interest to the news media.[60]

Many post-war visitors appear to have made the trip to Peckham as a result of their reading, one of the main sources of inspiration being *Health the Unknown*, a 1947 book by journalist John Comerford. He made no secret of the fact that his publication was intended to provide an (even more) popular version of *The Peckham Experiment* – quite free of criticism, as already noted at the time.[61] In terms of content the book differed very little from its template. But it contributed to the latter's credibility by seemingly confirming the centre's impact through an outsider's authentic testimony. In his book Comerford relates that he had already written its first chapters during the war and had then visited the reopened centre in the spring of 1946, quite prepared for disappointment. The investigations for his book, he explains, rapidly turned into a self-experiment. Comerford recapitulates how, during a stroll through the building – contrary to his normal behaviour – he had chatted uninhibitedly with the people he encountered there. He had been bitten by the centre bug, noting changes in himself that laid bare his own potential for optimization. He had, he went on, returned to the centre on one occasion, bringing along his own family to see what would happen. His children were thrilled by the centre, while he himself had soon developed a receptivity to the "whole pattern" of centre life.[62]

After the war the centre's presence in the press increased substantially. Tellingly – when it comes to the role it had come to play for its operators – we can trace this presence in great detail with the help of eight meticulously maintained books of cuttings.[63] They show that the overwhelming majority of reports on the centre appeared not in the specialist press but in the daily newspapers,[64] where it was often interpreted as a leisure centre for workers, indeed as a cheap holiday destination, a "shilling riviera".[65] It was also mentioned in the gossip columns, which reported, for example, on the premiere of *The Centre* – its first showing attended by Prime Minister Clement Attlee and Queen Mary in July 1948, in a Peckham cinema rented out especially for the occasion.[66] A visit by socially engaged actor Johnny Weissmüller, star of the *Tarzan* movies, was also noted.[67] Finally, the South London local press published many brief reports on new year's parties at the PHC, its anniversaries and the local stars of the Peckham film.

That the centre enjoyed such renown, attracting hordes of visitors, was due in no small part to Pearse's and Scott Williamson's extensive lecturing activities. These too were recorded precisely. Before the centre had even reopened the two directors had given dozens of talks in London, but also in further-flung parts of the country, at both state institutions and private debating clubs: the Eugenics Society, the Staff Luncheon Club of the Ministry of Health, the Royal College of Nursing, the Science Research Society, the British Federation of Social Workers, the SMA and the British Council Social Welfare Club, and even at obscure organizations such as the Anglo-Soviet Group in Swansea. Peckham was presented to students of the social sciences at the University of Edinburgh, various Rotary Clubs, teachers' associations, to policemen and RAF officers, and of course audiences in longstanding reformist institutions such as Bloomsbury House, as well as administrators from Welwyn Garden City, members of county councils throughout England and Scotland, Quaker meetings, local Labour clubs and local branches of the Fabian Society.[68]

After the war the two directors increasingly lectured abroad. At times, they were on the road for weeks; this too suggests that now they essentially used the centre as a showpiece rather than a generator or testing ground for their theories. Before 1945 was out, Pearse had travelled to Northern Ireland, where she spoke before the staff of welfare agencies, schools and hospitals. The same year, at the behest of the War Office's education division, she went on a reading tour for soldiers in the Middle East and shortly afterwards, funded by the British Council, to the Netherlands.[69] In 1949 she travelled to Paris, where the film about the centre was shown at the British ambassador's instigation, and to Villard-de-Lans, where the British Council arranged a photographic exhibition on the topic.[70] Perhaps the greatest coup, however, was the trip undertaken by the two centre directors to the east coast of the United States the previous year. Pearse spoke at the Community Service Society of New York and the medical faculties of Harvard, Yale and Johns Hopkins Universities. More impressive still, on March 16, 1948, in Lake Success, New York, Scott Williamson had the opportunity to talk before several hundred delegates of the General Assembly of the United Nations (UN), after a showing of *The Centre*.[71]

"Peckham" in the world's press

By the late 1940s the story of the Peckham Experiment had caught the attention of media across the world. It comes as no surprise that the centre cropped up particularly often in the press of the Commonwealth countries: Canadian newspapers had already reported on the opening of the original centre, while their coverage of its reopening was mirrored in the South African and New Zealand press.[72] *The Peckham Experiment* was discussed in India and Ceylon (Sri Lanka), in the *Palestine Post* and *Melbourne Age*.[73] After a visit to London, Dr E. Sanleralli, head of Trinidad's health service, immediately called for "periodic [national] overhaul plans".[74] But the centre was often mentioned in US print media as well.[75] It is striking that here its field of research was regarded as sociological rather than biological.[76] *The American Catholic Sociological Review*, however, considered the directors' natural scientific aspirations insignificant in light of the "spiritual principles" the centre was so clearly upholding.[77]

Examination of the (far rarer) German-language press reports reveals another, quite specific context of reception. By 1938 Hugh Jones had provided the *Wiener Tag* and *Basler Nachrichten* with a brief, matter-of-fact report on the "Peckham health club"; in 1936 the *Deutsche Medizinische Wochenschrift*, meanwhile, painted a wholly distorted picture of the centre, which comes across as a strictly organized hospital: a "cadre of doctors oversees everything."[78] Otherwise the project was absent from the press of Nazi Germany. Conversely, the periodicals catering to German expatriates in the United States and elsewhere frequently discussed the "contagious health" seemingly observable in Peckham.[79] Generally speaking, German-language publications mostly thought "Peckham" worth mentioning as a curiosity – as a "sanatorium for the healthy" or "school of health".[80]

A look at Sweden might help bring out how differently the London project could be perceived – even by participants in the same national debate. City planner Otto Danneskiöld-Samsøe was sent to Britain in 1945 to reconnoitre its planning culture. He was so fascinated by the centre that in 1949 he devoted an essay to it in *Byggmästaren*, Sweden's leading architectural journal. First and foremost, what he perceived in the centre was a method for overcoming "the modern person's difficulties in adapting to social planning", with the family enabling this process of adaptation.[81] Shortly before, Alva Myrdal had visited Peckham as well. With the arrogance of one of the leading social reformers in a country that appeared to be developing a "third way" between capitalism and socialism, she decided that this British experiment was worth emulating, even in "Sweden, the laboratory of future society". Unlike Danneskiöld-Samsøe, however, Myrdal regarded the centre as an attempt to provide every resident of a particular administrative district with a routine (social) medical examination, thus enhancing their "working efficiency".[82]

In fact the lecture tours, the film and the other forms of marketing appear to have aroused a desire for a similar centre in many places. For example, the idea of establishing a "Peckham" in Madras (Chennai) was aired on a number of occasions; following Pearse's lecture in New York a group was established with the goal of opening a centre there.[83] For the most part, however, these projects – grass-roots initiatives that as such must have been a source of pleasure to the two directors – failed to get beyond the establishment of various associations.[84] Only in South Africa did institutions inspired by the Peckham Experiment come to fruition.[85] In 1940 the Pholela Health Centre opened in a rural "native reserve" in Zulu-speaking south-western Natal. As in London there were periodic medical examinations and, it is claimed, members soon came to regard the staff as friends.[86] Conversely, the Fordsburg Community Health Centre, which was founded by the University of Johannesburg, provided basic medical care and was at the same time intended as a research, leisure and advisory centre. It was meant to help overcome the isolation and passivity of workers, with staff members avoiding any "'preaching' attitude".[87] Strikingly, only "Europeans" could take up membership of the Fordsburg centre, according to an article that included a map of the planned roll-out of further health centres in Johannesburg – in the "white" areas of the city only. It is disconcerting to note how participatory hopes go hand in hand here with the sociospatial segregation of "races".

Clearly, the Peckham legend was compatible with the most extraordinary range of visions of a better life across the world.

Notes

1   Annual Reports 1938/39, WL, SA/PHC/A.2/11, 18.
2   "Peckham Health Centre", *Medical Officer* (July 1940).
3   F.J. Osborn to W.R. Childs, June 19, 1945, TNA, AVIA 9/91.
4   The Pioneer Health Centre, 1941, WL, SA/PHC/B.4/8/3.
5   Mathew Reed, *Rebels for the Soil: The Rise of the Global Organic Food and Farming Movement* (London: Earthscan, 2010), 39–41; and Philip Conford, *The Origins of the Organic Movement* (Edinburgh: Floris Books, 2001). In the late 1940s and early 1950s Scott Williamson was co-editor of the Soil Association magazine, in which he published occasional book reviews and one article: George Scott Williamson, "What is Science?", *Mother Earth* 6, no. 4 (1952): 39–44. Mary Langman was to take charge of the farm after the war. She was one of the founders of the first wholefood shop on London's Baker Street in the early 1960s: "Mary Langman. Pioneering spirit who helped launch the wholefood movement", www.theguardian.com/news/2004/apr/26/guardianobituaries.food (accessed December 17, 2017).
6   Papers on Centre Home Farm at Oakley House, with notes on evacuation scheme, 1940, WL, SA/PHC/B.4/1.
7   Emergency Evacuation Plan, 1939, WL, SA/PHC/B.3/2.
8   War and the Family by Innes Pearse and Lucy Crocker, 1940, WL, SA/PHC/B.4/8/1.
9   *British Medical Journal* (August 3, 1940): 165.
10   E.N. Strong to Pearse, March 20, 1940, TNA, ED 102/2.
11   Memo on the Farm, undated, WL, SA/PHC/B.4/1.
12   Monica Pearson, "The Peckham Experiment: A Pioneer British Health Center", *The Social Service Review* 21 (1947): 134.
13   Daniel Ritschel, *The Politics of Planning. The Debate on Economic Planning in Britain in the 1930s* (Oxford: Clarendon, 1997), 144–183; Lewis and Brookes, *The Peckham Health Centre.*
14   An Enquiry into the State of Medical Practice. Document summarising the views of Dr. Williamson of the Pioneer Health Centre, May 27, 1935, LSE, PEP/WG/15/1.
15   Minutes of a meeting between the Health Group and Social Services Group, May 1, 1936, LSE, PEP/WG/15/1.
16   Minutes, Health Group, October 7, 1936, LSE, PEP/WG/15/3, 3.
17   Minutes, Health Group, February 1, 1937, LSE, PEP/WG/15/3.
18   The Pioneer Health Centre Peckham, October 20, 1937, LSE, PEP/WG/15/6; *Planning. A Broadsheet issued by PEP* (1944), 12–14.
19   Memorandum on the preparation of the Report on the British Health Services, undated [1937], LSE, PEP/WG/15/6, 1, 2–3.
20   On the history of the NHS, see esp. Charles Webster, *The National Health Service: A Political History* (Oxford: Oxford University Press, 1998).
21   (Memo) to Hendrion: The Pioneer Health Centre and the Polyclinics called "Health Centres" in the Proposals of the British Medical Association, May 24, 1943, WL, SA/PHC/B.4/6/1.
22   *A National Health Service. Ministry of Health. Department of Health for Scotland. Presented by the Minister of Health and the Secretary of State for Scotland to Parliament by Command of His Majesty* (London: Ministry of Health, 1944).
23   Draft letter, 1948, WL, SA/PHC/B.5/16/2.
24   "What Experts are Saying about the Health Plan", *News Chronicle* (February 18, 1944).

25 Draft letter on Questionnaire to BMJ, March 14, 1944, WL, SA/PHC/B.4/6/3.

26 Horder highlighted the importance of "positive health" in debates on housing and nutrition (*Hansard* 129, October 26, 1943), reconstruction (*Hansard* 130, October 9, 1943) and agriculture and health (*Hansard* 130, February 17, 1944). Soon afterwards, in a personal letter, R.P. Winfrey of the Halley Stewart Trust also attempted to persuade his old friend Willink of the importance of health centres of the Peckham type – partly by reminding him of their past foxhunting exploits: Winfrey to Willink, February 29, 1944, WL, SA/PHC/B.4/5/2.

27 Scott Williamson to Lord Geddes, January 30, 1944, WL, SA/PHC/B.4/6/2.

28 Scott Williamson, *Physician, heal thyself*, 50, 60.

29 Ibid., 129.

30 Ibid. Quotations: 124, 52, 109, 89, 115.

31 On the position of the medical profession within the debate on health, see Sharon Schildein Grimes, *The British National Health Service. State Intervention in the Medical Marketplace, 1911–1948* (London: Routledge, 1991).

32 Stewart, "For a Healthy London". However, Somerville Hastings, who was both committee chairman and involved in the SMA, had some positive things to say about Scott Williamson's centre: Somerville Hastings, "Health Centres", *Comrade* (October 1946).

33 *Medical Officer* (July 1945).

34 "A Revolutionary Scheme of Local Government", *British Medical Journal* (June 30, 1945): 911; "Health for all", *Tribune* (September 7, 1945).

35 L.J. Witts, "Physician, heal thyself", *Oxford Mail* (July 10, 1945).

36 Letter in answer to (Prof. L.J.) Witts's article in *Oxford Mail*, 1945, WL, SA/PHC/B.4/6/7.

37 Scott Williamson to Winfrey, January 5, 1945, WL, SA/PHC/B.4/5/2.

38 Pearse to Winfrey, December 7, 1942, WL, SA/PHC/B.4/5/1.

39 Several hundred copies of the first edition were distributed to the press and influential individuals (of a total of 2,000: Mary Gowing to Pearse, October 1, 1943, WL, SA/PHC/B.4/5/1). The minutes of a strategy meeting shortly before publication show what a broad readership the directors hoped the book would reach. For example, one topic of discussion was how best to access the "women's press" (Notes on Meeting for Mr. Sainsbury, January 21, 1943, WL, SA/PHC/B.4/5/1). The authors and publishers had given a lot of thought to the book's title, plumping for *The Peckham Experiment* as part of their advertising strategy: they were keen to use a name associated with an established reputation. Previously they had discussed a more anthropological proposal: "Man in the Making": Winfrey to Stanley Unwin, January 1, 1945, WL, SA/PHC/B.4/5/1.

40 See for example the volume published as part of the "Target of Tomorrow" series edited by Huxley, Beveridge and nutritional scientist Boyd Orr: James Mackintosh, *The Nation's Health* (London: Pilot Press, 1944), 23–27.

41 *The National Insurance Gazette* (January 27, 1944): 39–41.

42 "Community of Families", *The Church Times* (February 11, 1944): 61.

43 *Peace News* (November 1944).

44 "Biological Aspects of Health. Biologists in Search of Material", *Nature* 142 (1938): 134–135; "Biologists In Search Of Material", *Industrial Welfare* (1938): 167; "Biologists In Search Of Material", *British Medical Journal* (June 18, 1938): 1312; "The Peckham Health Centre. A Three-Years Survey", *British Medical Journal* (June 11, 1938): 1056–1057.

45 Rosa Ford, "The Peckham Health Centre. A record of pioneer work in building up positive health", *Nursing Times* (February 2, 1948): 148–151; "Family Health", *The Lancet* (March 3, 1946): 355; "The Peckham Experiment", *The Medical Officer* (January 1, 1944); M.J. Elsas, "The Peckham experiment: a study of the living structure of society", *Eugenics Review* 36, no. 1 (1944): 31–32.

46 Innes Hope Pearse, "Positive Health", *British Medical Journal* (July 18, 1942): 78–79; Innes H. Pearse "What is a Health Centre?", *Public Health* (November 1944): 15–18; Innes H. Pearse, "The Peckham Experiment", *Eugenics Review* 37, no. 2 (1945): 48–55; Mary Gowing, "Incentives to Parenthood. Some Data from the Pioneer Health Centre, Peckham", *Eugenics Review* 35, no. 2 (1943): 39–41.
47 Memo to Halley Stewart Trust, 1943, WL, SA/PHC/B.4/4/1.
48 Mary Langman, Some notes on the implications of the Peckham experiment, June 1986, WL, SA/PHC/C.13.
49 Notes of Meeting, February 27, 1945, WL, SA/PHC/B.4/4/3.
50 "The story of the 500", *Peckham* (May 1949), 7, WL, SA/PHC/B.5/22.
51 A petition on a matter of national and local importance, 1946, TNA, AVIA 9/91.
52 Notes of Meeting, February 27, 1945, WL, SA/PHC/B.4/4/3.
53 Circular Letter to the Subscribers, 1946, WL, SA/PHC/B.5/2.
54 The re-opening of the Pioneer Health Centre, Peckham on March 23rd 1946, WL, SA/PHC/B.5/23/1.
55 Innes Hope Pearse, Re-opening findings 1947–1951, WL, SA/PHC/B.5/11.
56 Mary Langman, G. S. W. and I. H. P. – approximate dates and places, 1983, WL, SA/PHC/C.13.
57 Scott Williamson to Trustees, July 9, 1946, WL, SA/PHC/B.5/15.
58 Record of Visitors, May–October 1949, WL, SA/PHC/B.5/9.
59 The Peckham Experiment – What Next?, 1947, WL, SA/PHC/B.5/20/3.
60 *The Observer* (March 13, 1949).
61 *The Times* (November 1, 1947).
62 John Comerford, *Health the Unknown. The Story of the Peckham Experiment* (London: Hamish Hamilton, 1947), 56–58, 60.
63 Cuttings books, WL, SA/PHC/A.3/1–8.
64 For the years 1933–1946 alone, a count reveals more than 70 mentions in *The Times* and its *Supplements*, ranging from brief to thorough reports. The *News Chronicle* discussed the centre 32 times, the *Daily Telegraph* 24, the *Daily Herald* 23, the *Observer* 22 and the *Daily Mirror* on 20 occasions.
65 *South London Press* (February 1, 1949).
66 Attlee to Scott Williamson, July 15, 1948, WL, SA/PHC/B.5/18/2. Queen Mary had already visited the centre before the war: Visit of HM Queen Mary, February 1939, WL, SA/PHC/B.3/19.
67 "'Tarzan' invited to health centre", *South London Observer* (February 13, 1948).
68 Lectures to Civilians, Lectures to Forces, WL, SA/PHC/B.4/3.
69 By 1944 the British Council had already acquired a large batch of *The Peckham Experiment* and it distributed the book across the world: Scott Williamson to Winfrey January 13, 1944, WL, SA/PHC/B.4/5/2.
70 "Taking Peckham to France", *Peckham* (June 1949), without page number, WL, SA/PHC/B.5/22.
71 American Itinerary, 1947, WL, SA/PHC/A.1/4; The Passing of Peckham, 1951, WL, SA/PHC/B.6/13. There are striking similarities between the definition of health already incorporated by the UN into the constitution of the World Health Organization in 1946 and certain premises informing the PHC researchers' work; this definition emphasized the holistic character of health and the importance of the environment to individual well-being: "Constitution of The World Health Organization", http://apps.who.int/gb/bd/PDF/bd47/EN/constitution-en.pdf?ua=1 (PDF, accessed December 17, 2017).
72 See for example J. Allen, "An Experiment in Health", *Health* 5, no. 1 (1937): 6–8; C.E.A. Bedwell, "With the Hospitals in Britain", *The Canadian Hospital* (May 1946): 500; "Experiment in Britain. Great Laboratory with Human Beings as Happy Subjects", *Montreal Daily Star* (May 3, 1947); "Peckham Health Centre",

Natal Mercury (January 7, 1946); John Hall, "Seeking a Secret", *Auckland Weekly News* (July 28, 1948).

73 "A New Approach to Public Health", *Times of India* (July 8, 1944); W.G. Wickremesinghe, "The Peckham Experiment", *The Ceylon Daily News* (April 24, 1947); "Biologist and Family get together", *Palestine Post* (June 2, 1944); "The Great Experiment. World Famous Centre", *Melbourne Age* (January 26, 1946).

74 "Family Club", *Trinidad Guardian* (May 19, 1946).

75 Bruno Gebhard, "The Peckham Experiment", *Medical Care* 4 (1944): 315–317; Arthur E. Morgan, "Elements of Community Life", *Community Service News* 2, no. 3 (1944): 1–4; Mary B. Palmer, "Experiment in Health", *Harpers Magazine* (May 1949): 327–432. Peckham was also mentioned in the *New York Herald Tribune* (April 18, 1947) and *Boston Post* (October 16, 1948).

76 "20 Years of Applied Sociology?", *Chicago Sun* (April 21, 1946); Maria Rogers, "The Peckham Experiment", *Sociometry* 8 (1945): 92–96; Pearson, "The Peckham Experiment"; Gordon W. Blackwell, "The Peckham Experiment", *American Sociological Review* 12 (1947): 259–260.

77 Jean F. Hewitt, "The Peckham Experiment", *The American Catholic Sociological Review* 7 (1946): 140.

78 Hugh Jones, "Gesundheitsclub von Peckham", *Wiener Tag* (January 19, 1938); *Basler Nachrichten* (January 27, 1938); "VI. Internationaler Kongreß für physikalische Therapie in London", *Deutsche Medizinische Wochenschrift* 29 (1936): 82.

79 "Ansteckende Gesundheit. Das englische 'Peckham Experiment'", *Aufbau* (January 21, 1944); P.E.M., "Ansteckende Gesundheit", *Argentinisches Tageblatt* (October 18, 1946).

80 "Vegetarier des Lebens. Ein Sanatorium für Gesunde – Der Krankheit den Krieg erklärt", *Telegraph* [Berlin] (July 16, 1949); "'Schule der Gesundheit' in London", *Schwäbische Volkszeitung* (August 10, 1949). In some post-war reports the influence of the "Third Reich" still makes itself felt. For example, a 1949 article in a Viennese newspaper applauds the fact that there are no "leaders" (Führer) at the centre. But the author then adds that what is astonishing is not so much "how much freedom members have here but the fact that they are capable of using this freedom". He goes on to express a desire to see the "breeding techniques" developed in London applied to Austria. Friedrich Katscher, "Das Experiment von Peckham", *Arbeiter-Zeitung* [Vienna] (February 2, 1949).

81 Otto Danneskiold-Samsøe, "Peckham-experimentet", *Byggmästaren* 28 (1949): 321.

82 Alva Myrdal, "Hälsan är fritidsnöje i PECKHAM", *Vi* 33, no. 34 (1946): 7.

83 According to a flyer on *The Centre*, 1948, WL, SA/PHC/B.5/18/1; see also "A Center for Health", *New York Herald-Tribune* (March 9, 1948).

84 This applied to an initiative launched by students and the city council in Cardiff and to the efforts of a group linked with the Fabian Society to establish a centre in Bury St Edmunds in Suffolk (Oliver Powell to Winfrey, July 26, 1945, WL, SA/PHC/B.4/5/2). The Peckham Experiment Propaganda Group for Oxford also came to grief (see *Oxford Times*, March 15, 1946). Plans for a community centre in Windsor based on the PHC (*Windsor Express*, January 31, 1947) fell by the wayside, as did the efforts made by former PHC staff member Kenneth Barlow to establish such a centre as the nucleus of a new residential complex near Coventry (see Chapter 13).

85 In the early 1940s – before Apartheid itself had taken off – the South African Ministry of Health planned a whole network of health centres reserved for different "racial groups": Anne Digby, *Diversity and Division in Medicine. Health Care in South Africa from the 1800s* (Oxford: Lang, 2006): 413–419.

86 *Biology and Human Affairs* 14 (1944): 5.

87 "Centre of Public Health. First Steps in a Practical Plan", *Libertas* (December 1943): 25.

10 "The Passing of Peckham" (1946–1959)

In the second half of the 1940s the Peckham Experiment was a boon to all involved. PHC members ultimately gained from the success of the scientists' publications, which generated the funds that allowed the centre to be reopened. The scientists, meanwhile, could pursue their biological mission across the world secure in the knowledge that back home in London there was a place that proved the legitimacy of their endeavours. This state of affairs, however, pertained for a few years at most. For the research at the centre increasingly took on the air of a self-fulfilling prophecy, attracting ever harsher criticism from outsiders. Following the reopening in 1946, in case of doubt staff members could read up on how they ought to envisage a natural order. To all appearances, in fact, getting a job at the centre required a willingness to adopt the directors' perspective on it. Curiously enough, this involved approaching it without a methodological toolkit. We get a sense of this from the internship report produced by sociology student Enid Mills, who worked as assistant to the curator for a few months in 1948. Mills wrote:

> The Centre allows [one] to observe the normal growth of a society in which the people have the opportunity to develop freely. The student comes expecting to observe, but soon realises that her greatest task is to discover how to observe. Natural growth being subtle, she finds in the Centre that it is woven of the hundred and one commonplace incidents of everyday life. The art of tracing the relevant amongst the irrelevant must be learnt, yet a sense of wholeness must be retained.[1]

For Mills this initially seems to amount to the typical intern's problem of an inadequate job description: "[T]he student is shown the building and left bewilderingly alone. On no account is she advised what to look for, where to look or how to look." What is truly interesting, however, are the reflections this lack of structure inspires in Mills. She arrives at the centre expecting to observe social health. But no one tells her what this looks like. She is left alone, and this sparks an awareness of her perceptual limits:

She [the student] becomes sharply aware that she is an individual and that this makes null and void her chances of observation. To observe, she must establish a relationship with the society of the Centre wherein lies the possibility of mutual exchange. She must become part of the Centre pattern. Having established herself as part of the Centre she has regained her individuality but now as one related to a whole. As a student, she is given the chance of fulfilling the double function of being in the pattern and aware of the pattern. Once she has learned how to observe, she becomes increasingly aware of the variety of her opportunities.[2]

Mills's participant (self-)observation has little in common with the ideal of an objective, scientific persona, one separated from the process or object observed with the aid of a methodology.[3] Yet this lack of objectivity was just what the directors favoured. They had begun to suggest to their employees that they open themselves to a sensory experience; they should anticipate and accept changes in their own behavioural patterns as part of the experiment. Pearse elucidated this in 1979 through a fictional dialogue between a member of staff and the directors: "'What are my duties as a member of the Social staff?' 'None: only go and "look".' The answer, if there is one, is *there*. [...] It won't be the one you are expecting."[4] Two decades earlier Scott Williamson had linked his staff members' suitability to their willingness to strip themselves of the aloof stance of the scientist. The centre's purpose, he wrote, had been "to provide a field of observation and education for both the scientists and their 'guinea-pigs'[; it is] in fact a mutual benefit association". He added: "The Centre staff [...] had to shed his or her authority that had been built up in their professional capacity of doctors, nurse, educationalist and social worker etc."[5] Little wonder, then, that some members of staff grew sceptical of scientific methods in general. Douglas Trotter, for example, the post-war curator we met earlier, later rejected the term "observer" entirely because it implied a hierarchy. Even the word "interpretation" displeased him: "[It] should be reserved to imply that the meaning is given with weight and authority."[6]

In the post-war period centre employees were frequently dismissed if they failed to fit in. This occurred at a point in time when Pearse and Scott Williamson were having trouble recruiting staff in the first place. In the 1970s Pearse recalled that just a few applicants had displayed the requisite "aspiration for adventure", which included a willingness to deal with users who saw themselves as co-researchers in the Peckham Experiment: "The members were ready to tell them what had to be done."[7]

Criticisms from within and without

It took an astonishingly long time for the first former staff member to express public criticisms. In 1948 Michael Chance, who had worked as head of the laboratory for a time, provided the first sceptical insider's view of the centre.[8]

Two years later he fleshed out his analysis in *The Lancet*. Here he highlighted the chasm between the centre's renown and the quality of its scientific output: "Scientists were quick to realise that the reporting of the scientific work lacked the standard of accuracy expected in scientific investigation." Conversely, he went on, many social workers and other essentially practice-oriented specialists had been enthusiastic about the centre – until they visited it: "Over and over again visitors [...] left entirely mystified, unable to take back to their friends any clear idea of what was being done." The centre had made a promising start as a project that initiated group activities on the assumption that these could prompt the "cooperation of the individual in his own cure".[9] However, he asserted, the directors had never seriously tackled the problem of how to describe the highly complex processes that had been induced at the centre in a valid, scientific manner. Quite the reverse in fact: lacking a thorough understanding of these processes, according to Chance they had influenced them in a wholly unsystematic way:

> Many investigators came to the Peckham Health Centre and asked where the discipline was, and they always received the answer that there was no discipline. If by this was meant that there were no principles by which people could understand what the limits of their freedom were, this statement is true. But members had only to try something that was disapproved of to find that definite limits were in fact set to social activity. [...] [T]he arbitrariness with which on occasion the staff interfered with the activities of the members was startling.

Chance indicates that he had tried in vain to talk to Pearse and Scott Williamson about the incoherence of their approach: "[L]acking serious and frank discussion it has been impossible to find out how to make sociological observations in these circumstances, nor have sociologists been asked to help."[10] Characteristically, Scott Williamson penned a reply that failed to address any of Chance's criticisms. Instead he imputed to the latter an inability to embrace the special research conditions in Peckham.[11]

It was not the first time the researchers had come under fire from their scientific peers. *The Peckham Experiment* had already inspired a good deal of scepticism. A review in *Nature* in 1944 was particularly hard-hitting: "It is difficult not to feel that their preconceived ideas about 'the living structure of society' stand in the way of the experimenters."[12] In much the same way as Chance, it went on to underline the profound difference between the social and scientific aspects of the centre's work. From a preventive medicine perspective, its value to its members was beyond dispute. The researchers' assessment of this value, however, left much to be desired: "[I]t would be a pity if further progress in such an important technique of medical research were prejudiced by their views and methods, which many people will find scientifically unacceptable." A year later we discern a certain exasperation in the *Medical Press*. In a sense Scott Williamson was too modest: "[H]e clearly bases his ideas on the way in which group activities developed at the Peckham Centre without taking into full account the way in which the personal influence of himself and his colleagues there, however unobtrusive, may have both guided and controlled."[13] What some regarded as a form of understatement, however, others saw as scientific malpractice. In the *Bulletin of Hygiene*, for example, community physician John Ryle pointed out that the Peckham researchers' admirable enthusiasm was not matched by usable findings, not least because of the questionable relationship between normativity and empirical knowledge at the centre: "Can an experiment which [...] addresses itself to the alteration of the conditions of life and health which it sets out to investigate be accepted as a basically sound experiment?"[14]

Finally, in 1950, a scathing retrospective on the centre as a whole by bacteriologist I.H. Winner appeared in the *Scientific Worker*. *The Peckham Experiment*, Winner contended, contained "numerous woolly statements about a variety of sociological topics which would not stand scientific examination". What is more, he went on, the book could have been written without reference to the centre: scientists had long been aware of the efficacy of medical interventions that incorporated the family environment. Above all, he asserted, not everyone was willing to be a guinea pig, diminishing the centre's representativity. This, he went on, did not delegitimize the research per se – but the researchers had failed completely to discuss these limitations.[15]

We might be tempted to explain the numerous criticisms of data collection at the centre in light of the dissemination and advance of statistical methods in medicine and the social sciences in the 1940s and early 1950s. This has often been viewed as the scientific correlate of the expansion of the welfare state after the Second World War, as the "politics of method".[16] Because the centre made a splash within political discourse, however, increasingly it was also scrutinized by socialists and feminists, who uniformly dismissed it as revisionist. In 1944, for example, sociologist Mark Benney (later colleague of US scholar of conformism David Riesman) discussed *The Peckham Experiment* in the *International Women's News*. People, according to Benney, must get used to the feeling of isolation in modern mass society. But many individuals, he went on, found this difficult, which explained the widespread longing for primordial, natural communities. Such wishful thinking being incompatible with its claims of verification, science had, Benney asserted, been spared this tendency – until now. For him *The Peckham Experiment* was an attempt to tear down this bastion of objectivity. The book contained "the most irritatingly placental balderdash that it ever has been my duty to read though". It was so "steeped and distorted in the authors' stream of fantasy that one hesitates to accept even the most respectable looking column of figures". The authors' scientific terminology, Benney contended, cloaked an alarming mysticism: "When scientific responsibility has been thrown over board so early in the book, it is not surprising to find social responsibilities following." As an example he pointed out that Pearse and Crocker regarded equality between the sexes as biologically risky. Anyone expounding such controversial ideas, Benney stated, should base them on more than just "predigested case-history". The book, he concluded, had "a natural place in the social programme of reaction". In fact, it was doubly dangerous: it might prompt "intelligent" people to discard even the positive lessons of the centre, while conservatives might regard it as providing scientific corroboration of their views.[17] A review of the new edition of *Biologists in Search of Material* in the bulletin of the SMA had already put forward similar arguments in 1947. The reviewer was pathologist David Stark Murray, who was to become president of the association a short time later and had some influence on the organization of the NHS. In recent times, he wrote, whenever health was up for discussion someone would assert that Peckham was the template to emulate. It had become difficult to say "no" to this. But the book, he went on, exuded a "patronising air". And given the authors' failure to consider economic issues one might define the "Peckham method" as follows: "working in a capitalist state and being very careful not to notice it."[18]

The directors' fall from power

In the summer of 1949 the centre was on the verge of bankruptcy, making it imperative to raise funds. Its financial backers, however, were concerned about its image in the scientific community, especially the Health Trust, which administered the centre's finances. In line with the aforementioned overall trend towards quantification in (social) medicine and the social sciences, the members of the Health Trust pushed for the appointment of a statistician in order to bolster the validity of the project's findings.[19] Their gradual loss of patience with the two directors is clearly apparent in a series of letters: "His [the statistician's] criticisms of the doctors will do what we want for the next stage. It will either condition them for research to come, or induce their resignation, without our having to force either."[20] In September the Health Trust requested that Scott Williamson and Pearse submit a proposal on the centre's future. As they had already done during the war, they proposed turning it into a pure research institute. The centre as it then was seems to have been quite ill-suited to their needs. The following year, they suggested, it should be closed.[21]

The Health Trust then tasked an external team of advisers, made up of renowned scientists, with evaluating Scott Williamson and Pearse's proposals.[22] Though the experts were well disposed towards the pair, they did not hesitate to highlight the discrepancy between the centre's scientific aspirations and normative goals, while conceding that in the social sciences (!) strict objectivity was a fundamentally problematic goal. Nonetheless they suggested investigating users' social background. (Why had *they* become members? What had stopped other people from taking up membership?) They also called for more detailed quantitative analysis of the "[c]hanges in social and spiritual values, changes in behavioural patterns, and changes in attitude and philosophy towards health" instigated by the experiment.[23] In their final report the experts welcomed the proposal to turn the centre into a research institute for human biology. However, in the spirit of the National Health Service Act, which had now come into force, what they meant by this was a health centre with an attached research institute. In concrete terms this would mean involving local general practitioners (GPs), in other words the centre would provide medical treatment as well. This would be made possible by mixed financing consisting of user fees and funds from the Ministry of Health, the MRC and LCC. None of those involved in the Health Trust were in any doubt that this meant stripping Scott Williamson and Pearse of their power: "It was obvious now that the new regime could not carry on as did the old one with a blank cheque to the Medical directors."[24] Some of the centre's longstanding supporters criticized this, though they tended to underline the moral obligation not to deprive Pearse and Scott Williamson of their life's work rather than highlighting their scientific achievements.[25]

In any case, the solution favoured by the funders and scientific advisers failed to spark the interest of the state institutions they had in mind. The centre closed in March 1950. The efforts of the MP for Camberwell, Wilfried Vernon, and appeals from centre users, some of them addressed directly to Aneurin Bevan, were in vain.[26] Their hand will not have been strengthened by Pearse's and Scott Williamson's repeated attacks on the health minister in previous years – though Bevan was in fact a keen exponent of experimental structures, who, among other things, championed the building of a health centre in Woodberry Down, North London, in 1948. Their criticisms might help explain Bevan's sardonic response to an enquiry in the House of Commons on the future of the centre: "MR. BEVAN said he would be delighted to receive from those who were in charge of the Peckham Health Centre any conclusions on the research aspects. So far as he knew, they had had no concrete conclusions."[27]

The money trail

So far the history of the centre's fall may seem tragic, the result of a scientific discovery the Peckham directors were ill-equipped to fully grasp. In addition, many commentators have asserted that the dirigist zeitgeist prevailing in the UK after the war meant the country itself was not yet ready for "Peckham". Pearse and Scott Williamson themselves put forward the latter interpretation in their obituary of the centre, the leaflet "The Passing of Peckham", which they dispatched to their supporters across the world in 1951.[28] Indeed, as we have seen, some critics of the experiment put its methodological shortcomings down to a conservative political agenda, emphasizing the precarious position it was in given the scientistic and egalitarian social policy mainstream of the time. While this did not equate to a death sentence, it did make it easier for people to distance themselves from the failing project.[29]

Yet several pieces of evidence indicate that there was more going on than just a shift in the political mood that altered the scientific and administrative conditions for initiatives such as the PHC. Certainly, the local authorities, on which such projects depended, had lost some of their powers to the NHS. But there was also a general waning of interest in the borderlands of biology and the social sphere, the hybrid field in which Scott Williamson might have found a sympathetic ear. Increasingly, medical research and funding institutions prioritized clinical experiments, a development closely correlated with the expansion of the system of NHS hospitals. The post-war focus on biomedicine, meanwhile, generally meant a technology-backed, laboratory-based science; beginning in the United States, this expedited the discipline's biochemical and genetic "molecularization". In parallel to this, pharmacology increasingly promised to wipe out illnesses entirely with the help of sulphonamide-based antibiotics and the seeming panacea of cortisone.[30] Taken together, these trends made expensive, commercially uninteresting programmes of preventive medicine seem outdated. Moreover, such programmes took a long time to have an effect and thus held out little prospect of the speedy successes health ministers liked to crow about.[31]

But there is one question I have left to one side so far. How did the centre become bankrupt in the first place? Oddly enough, those who championed the resurrection of "Peckham" failed to address the economics of the PHC, in other words the very aspect that would presumably have been most worth discussing when it came to the project's repeatability. The books written by the Peckham researchers also have very little to say about money. By way of contrast, the archival material provides eloquent testimony on the topic. The number of surviving documents on experimental practices is meagre compared with the mass of funding applications and calls for donations addressed to organizations like the Carnegie Trust and Rockefeller Foundation, insurance companies, industrialists and the British nobility.

As we saw earlier, when it was launched in the mid 1920s one of the main functions of the experiment was as an economic pilot project. It was intended to prove that a comprehensive form of health care was possible without state subsidies or administration. Centre members were granted increasing freedoms (the effects of which the researchers then began to regard as natural phenomena) partly in the hope that this would attract more users and thus generate more income. Such hopes were dashed. The centre on St Mary's Road remained dependent on charity, which the directors regarded as no less harmful than large-scale redistribution.

In fact, as early as 1933, several years before the opening of the centre on St Mary's Road, state agencies were already expressing doubts about its prospects of success. When Scott Williamson and his colleagues attempted to attain the sponsorship of Lucy Baldwin, wife of de facto Prime Minister Stanley Baldwin, she asked the Ministry of Health for information on the project. It advised against sponsorship. In terms of medical services, the Ministry claimed, the centre was superfluous; it merely reduplicated the work of other institutions.[32] Not long afterwards Ewen Montagu contacted Minister of Health Hilton Young in person requesting his support.[33] The latter commissioned a detailed report on the centre, which came to a similar conclusion. A discussion with the medical officer of health in Camberwell, the report stated, had shown the project in a poor light. He viewed it as a second attempt at an experiment that had already failed once. He was sceptical about the new centre's prospects of financing itself: "[H]e does not consider from the experience of the first Centre that they are likely to be successful administrators from a financial standpoint."[34]

The fact that it took five years after the closure of its predecessor project for the new centre to be inaugurated was due to difficulties obtaining funds. The construction of the building itself became a realistic prospect only after Jack Donaldson had donated half his inheritance.[35] Nevertheless, between 1935 and 1939 the centre then rapidly got into debt. By 1937 it already had a huge overdraft.[36] At times the cafeteria lost so much money that the directors considered reducing its staff in order to keep its prices affordable.[37] In 1939, on the General Committee, for the first time Maureen Stanley proposed dropping the idea of autonomy entirely while also suggesting that the directors cease their attacks on the medical authorities.[38] The official report for the same year then openly admitted that in the near future user fees were very unlikely to cover running costs. Increasing the fees, however, was out of the question. The report also stated that the centre's catchment area had been enlarged by a factor of five, in other words an attempt had been made to attract members in an area home to 25,000 families, but without success: just 5% of contacted Peckham residents had visited the centre, while only 2% of potential new member families had joined.[39] This must have been deeply exasperating: the step roundly contradicted the claim, still being made around this time, that the centre was worth preserving because of its sample, selected according to strictly scientific criteria.[40]

In May 1939 Scott Williamson performed a volte face, soliciting the support of Edward Mellanby, secretary of the MRC, which had earlier financed his thyroid research. Mellanby asked him for a statement on the centre's research findings, which he then forwarded to Bradford Hill of the London School of Hygiene for assessment, remarking:

> [F]rom the point of view of accumulation of data they are completely snowed under. It may be that they have got a lot of valuable stuff there which will be wasted because of their inability to classify and publish their work. On the other hand the work may be of such a nature that it can lead nowhere from a scientific point of view.[41]

Hill, himself a statistician, soon replied that he had visited the centre and borrowed a dozen family files so he could look them over at his leisure. They had been unreadable, the data collected unsystematically: certain individuals had been constantly examined, others barely at all. It would, of course, be possible to help out with the analysis of this data; but he had the impression that Scott Williamson had no interest in this. He was concerned solely to obtain "financial support to enable the place to keep running – I believe it is on the rocks".[42] Mellanby's subsequent replies to Scott Williamson were evasive, prompting him to (temporarily) adopt a defensive tone. Scott Williamson wrote to Hill:

> Our examinations and methods have only now become standardised, so that looking over past notes means shifting the point of view several times. [...] [W]e have been groping in the dark for three years and are only now coming out into the light.[43]

Apparently the centre avoided bankruptcy solely due to the outbreak of war.[44] Pearse and Scott Williamson later propagated the myth that the war had thwarted the experiment before it could demonstrate its long-term impact (in an economic sense). However, they had to admit that the sequestration of the building, which the state rented for a time in the early 1940s, had helped pay off some of its debts.[45]

After its reopening in 1946 an attempt was made to place the centre's finances on a firmer footing. Ownership of the property was transferred to the aforementioned Health Trust – a legal construct founded by the directors and some of the centre's sponsors, most prominently the Halley Stewart Trust, which had helped finance the reopening of the centre. The Health Trust then rented the building and land to its operators for a symbolic sum. While this relieved some of Pearse and Scott Williamson's burdens, it also shifted power away from them. In the shape of Donald Wilson the centre took on a general manager and, after consulting with the users, doubled the membership fee to two shillings.[46] Nonetheless the situation worsened again rapidly, a growing source of frustration to the members of the Health Trust. Even the major donation from South Africa received the following year on the initiative of Jan Smuts failed to resolve the crisis. In 1948 a newly established finance committee then discussed, for the first time, the centre's integration into the NHS.[47]

It is in this context that the criticisms of the centre's methodology became a real problem. For instance, the fact that many state institutions were no longer as well disposed towards the centre as they had been before the war seems to have contributed to the Health Trust's decision to – at least partly – dissociate itself from Pearse and Scott Williamson. When the Trust contacted J.A. Charles of the Ministry of Health in order to gain its support, once again he asked Mellanby for his opinion on the centre's merits.[48] But Mellanby merely recapitulated how disorderly the files had been in 1939.[49]

In February 1949 the centre's accounts were once again in the red, to the tune of £23,000.[50] In December, when the Health Trust pressed for the centre's reconceptualization – probably partly in an attempt to prevent at least some of the invested funds from being seized by the banks – its closure date had already been fixed: March 31, 1950.[51] Earlier there had been unsuccessful talks with the LCC about selling the centre. The council had made it clear that as owner, it would open the centre's doors to all interested parties, not just families and residents of the district, something the trust rejected.[52] In July 1950, however, the LCC acquired the centre anyway, without specifying how it would be used. The only condition was that it could not continue to use the name "Pioneer Health Centre",[53] enabling Scott Williamson and Pearse to copyright the Peckham legend. The Health Trust agreed a price of £57,000 for building and land and a further £3,000 for furniture and equipment.[54] When the debts had been cleared there was £20,000 left over, a sum that was converted into scholarships for Scott Williamson and Pearse; in this sense, they undoubtedly benefited from the winding-up of the centre.[55]

Within the LCC the purchase provoked a heated debate because it was unclear how the premises might actually be used.[56] One critic warned: "The Minister [of Health] has twice indicated to the Council that this building is a white elephant."[57] Previously a Conservative MP for Peckham had campaigned for the centre's membership criteria to be retained.[58] It almost appears as though – with the Peckham Experiment continuing to attract a great deal of attention in the media – the LCC came under pressure to associate itself with the old centre. In any event, after the signing of the contract it was announced that the new centre would feature a nursery and a research department, while parts of the building would be used as an evening school. Only the first floor would be reserved for the local GPs.[59] In the meantime Pearse and Scott Williamson had begun to assail the welfare state in general and the LCC in particular, accusing the latter of feigning interest in resuming the experiment.[60]

From guinea pigs to citizens' group

Directors, trustees and the LCC decided the centre's fate over the heads of users. While Scott Williamson and Pearse informed them of developments, they presented them in the form of a fait accompli. In February 1950 Scott Williamson discussed the impending closure in the last of his Sunday talks. He seemed depressed and rueful: "I think we made an error there, in that we could not anticipate that the whole trend of thought was turning from voluntary private support to the compulsory principle." But he said nothing about the reasons for the centre's dependency on external cash injections or the scientific criticisms of the centre. Nor did he address his longstanding goal of continuing to convert it from a welfare centre into a research unit. When the members in attendance – including Ron Goldsmith and Elsie Purser – offered to establish a committee to assess potential savings by users, Scott Williamson went into lecturing mode. He reminded them that one of the key research topics had been the growth of "responsibility within a community". A savings committee, however, would represent a form of institutionalization that would impede this growth. He would rather end the research project, he hinted, than be forced to make scientific compromises. A contribution by Amy Moor articulates genuine veneration for Scott Williamson but also reveals his tremendous interpretive power:

> I want to say something to the doctors. Peckham has become my life. I know that if it is humanly possible for the Doctors to keep the Centre open they will do it. because [sic] Dr Williamson is not only a pure scientist but one of the most human and loving of men, I only hope that he will not be tempted to keep the Centre open on any terms but the best – which means that he will have free control of the Centre (applause).[61]

Before 1949 was over, the PHC Members Association had been founded. After the centre's closure the activists involved in the association saved up the membership fees they would have paid for use of the centre and rented rooms in the neighbouring building, which they used as their headquarters as they protested against the closure. When it transpired that the LCC was planning to make the centre a theme of its exhibition at the 1951 Festival of Britain, they threatened to hand out leaflets at the entrance pointing out that the original experiment had been wound up.[62] The members association aroused some interest when it announced the holding of a demonstration in Trafalgar Square, though it was later cancelled.[63] The users managed to arrange a meeting with female MPs on March 23, 1950; according to the minutes, they were sympathetic to their cause.[64] Conversely, the users' delegation felt that a number of London parliamentarians with whom they subsequently met had been deliberately intimidating. They had been furious with these politicians at the time, as Purser recalled in 1989. She was probably correct in her assumption that they tended to sneer at the revolt of the Peckham neighbours.[65] What she failed to realize, however, was that the ex-members were dealing with institutions that simply believed them to be defending a privilege.[66] Funding the centre with public money while retaining its exclusive conditions of admission would have meant directly subsidizing a very small part of London's population. The LCC at least would scarcely have been able to justify this.

Many years later Purser described a visit to the Queen's Road Health Centre, the new name of the institution opened in 1952 under the aegis of the LCC. One scene in particular stuck in her memory:

> A teenager came and stood behind one of the pillars watching the [dancing] class. He was doing no harm at all, but the Area Principal came along, and the teenager was told off and made to look small. Had it been Centre days, he would have been nicely ignored, or smiled at, and he could have watched at any time he liked.

Something that had been encouraged in the old centre, as a form of interest in others that was conducive to activity, was now punished as voyeurism.

Purser proved herself an eager disciple of Pearse and Scott Williamson when she demonstrated through another example why, under its new leadership, the centre had a demotivating effect:

> We had to join a swimming class, otherwise we couldn't use the pool; so we did. I think it lasted about three evenings, we were just so bored. We didn't want at our age to compete in the Olympics – just to swim – but, as soon as we fell out of line, we were told to get into place.[67]

In fact the new institution was something of a problem child. While the evening school attracted students, the plan for researchers to use part of the building was put on ice. When plans were hatched in 1955 to turn the build-ing into a medical centre, the established local doctors protested.[68] None-theless, in 1959 alterations were made to the building; it was equipped with a lift and an X-ray installation and was reopened in 1961 as the South East London General Practitioners' Centre. Doctors from all over London could now make use of the building's equipment with negligible administrative effort.[69] By now the members association had wound up. A kindergarten it had been running was closed in August 1956 due to lack of interest.

Proof of the pudding

The experiment was over. Before turning to the way the ideas it generated rumbled on beneath the surface, it is helpful to go into a bit more detail about Scott Williamson's rather unusual post-war style of thought. My goal here is to elucidate how selective the perception of his theories has been. Scott Williamson's resistance to criticism appears to have had much to do with his role at the centre: he tended to surround himself with people who were prepared to accept his interpretive power, turning the building on St Mary's Road into something of an echo chamber by the 1940s at the latest. This setting bolstered the resonance of his ideas but was increasingly impervious to external criticisms. Furthermore, this sequestering process reinforced his tendency to ensconce himself within his own theoretical framework. His col-leagues at least regarded him as the embodiment of the process of biological and social synthesis cultivated at the centre. For these reasons, at the very moment when outsiders began to take a closer look at practices in the centre, Scott Williamson refused to contemplate his status as sole authority within a "laboratory of anarchism". Even those sympathetic to qualitative research must have perceived something almost alchemical in his apparent belief that he had come across a theory somehow explaining life itself, yet one only he himself could "prove". By 1950, Julian Huxley, for example, was no longer much convinced by Scott Williamson's research. The latter had previously sent him an article he wished to publish in the *Journal of Experimental Biology*. Huxley saw no prospect of this happening:

> So much of your thinking is expressed in terms which are really mere analogies, rather than based on scientific knowledge; an [sic] personally, I am always put off by a lot of new terminology and also by attempts at over-sweeping generalisation such as you indulge in. My recollection is that you have plenty of material to do this – e. g. pointing out the value of freedom of choice, of working through a family group etc.[70]

In the 1930s Huxley himself had still been partial to normative readings of the evolutionary process of progressive differentiation. In his widely read book *Evolution: The Modern Synthesis* (1942), conversely, he had defined evolution emphatically as non-purposeful. Hence, in another letter to Scott Williamson he wrote: "To say that [evolution] is a 'force' seems to me the most dangerous and misleading kind of vitalistic mysticism, which at all costs is to be avoided in biology."[71]

In the early 1950s Scott Williamson was isolated, partly because of his refusal to accept the complexity of the factors that had brought his experiment to an end – and as a result of his uncoordinated attacks on peculiarly abstract opponents. Mary Langman may also have been on to something. Conceding that Scott Williamson showed less and less intellectual flexibility in the last few years of his life, she explained that "he was old and tired".[72] Among his colleagues in the medical profession he could no longer slough off the stigma of the charlatan. When Scott Williamson died in 1953, a sensitive obituary in *The Lancet* dealt almost exclusively with doubts about the centre's scientific value.[73]

As evident in his critics' statements, one tendency in particular demonstrates how far Scott Williamson had ultimately distanced himself from contemporary scientific standards: his evaluation of statistics. In 1929 he was still stating that "continuity of observation" was of the utmost importance if "the inquiry [was] to be a scientific and statistical one".[74] It was not long, however, before the Peckham researchers' texts began to aggressively dismiss the possibility of backing up their observations with figures. By 1936 Scott Williamson had come to regard statistics as a perspective that was prone both to getting lost in details and to constructing overly simplistic causalities. To him, it had in fact itself become a symptom of undesirable social developments within mass society, which could only be remedied by deploying a "different mathematic".[75] When the project had folded he wrote to Jack Donaldson that the Peckham researchers had probably been too far ahead of their time to be understood: "Perhaps this is my fault for diving into a deep-end – before I had got the information for some of my theories."[76] In a 1951 letter to R.P. Winfrey, however, he indicated that those aspects others had criticized as metaphysical fairy tales had been obvious to those who had experienced them: "The proof of the pudding is in the Eating not in the Statistics of the pudding."[77] A few lines later he compared himself with Isaac Newton.[78]

As progressive as Scott Williamson's personal habitus seems, his thinking tended to stumble backwards rather than forwards. In the 1940s he abandoned himself to an ever more extravagant linguistic frenzy. Imagery became argument, while words took on idiosyncratic meanings, at times descending into contradictory metaphors. He coined peculiar neologisms and put forward intricate definitions that camouflaged an essentially tauto-logical proposition: life is explicable in terms of its vitality. This applies especially to a series of draft chapters written during the war for a planned major theoretical work. Here Scott Williamson viewed the centre as a dockyard that repaired human ships, enabling them to obtain the A1 clas-sification in Lloyd's *Register of Shipping*; in this context he viewed himself as a "biological engineer".[79] The natural world – as he sought to prove with ruminations on bipolarity (of eyes and genders) – obeys a dialectical principle of growth, though this was in need of revival. This required a return to innocence, something Scott Williamson believed to be present in the "man-in-the-street" and "woman-in-the-home", whom he contrasted with the "man-in-the-know", an ignorant cynic and monopolist. Feeling rather than rationality is the pilot of the human machine; planning is a form of hubris, because every natural phenomenon is cast into the contingent "stream of life".[80] Rather than modern boats that carry energy with them, unwaveringly following routes laid down in advance, it is the sailing ship that embodies the ideal way of life, because it uses "emergy [sic] [...]: the power of Circumstance." The human being must learn to nimbly exploit this "emergent" energy of the context, to take the helm, to turn off the auto-matic controls.[81] Scott Williamson's evidence of the decline in people's abil-ity to make use of this "emergy" comes in the form of linguistic observations: he cites the fact that in Oxfordshire dialect the word "rails" sounds like the word "rules".[82] Even when trying to prove his point that prescription and authority are pathological, he resorts to punning: rather than "warming" the body, a guiding light merely provides a "warning".[83] At times we are left with the feeling that he was playing linguistic games without really knowing what he wanted to say.

As mentioned above, although it was planned as the second part of *The Peckham Experiment*,[84] his great synthesis was never completed. The text published posthumously in 1965 under the title *Science, Synthesis, and Sanity. An Inquiry into the Nature of Living*, was a collage, painstakingly assembled by Pearse from a mass of texts, ranging from scribbled notes to finished chapters.[85] To attempt to convey the contents of this book in detail would merely be to create the same kind of florilegium. We are presented with sev-eral hundred pages characterized by extreme redundancy. Here the Peckham Experiment is merely the trigger for a meandering line of argument, which no longer has – or seeks to have – any connection with any kind of medical problematic and never mentions other research. The title itself privileges the play of language over precision: the term "sanity" seldom crops up in the text; clearly the alliteration was just too tempting.

The book was a flop. A number of reviews appeared, which often praised the text's originality but focused chiefly on the PHC.[86] A review in the *New*

Scientist imputed to Scott Williamson a talent for inventing new words for philosophical truisms, making fun of his "do it yourself approach to the whole range of semantics".[87] Another reviewer merely thought the author confused.[88]

Probably due to this experience, Pearse herself was rather cautious in *The Quality of Life* when discussing the verifiability of her observations. Still, she did not refrain from using terms such as "experiment" and "scientific", just as the book's subtitle, *The Peckham Approach to Human Ethology*, implied that it was a contribution to behavioural science. (The main title was evidently Pearse's attempt to interface with the "quality of life" discourses so prevalent in the 1970s.) The book even includes a section entitled "the observation of wholes". This sounds like a discussion of methodology but is quite the opposite: wholes cannot be "recorded", to cite the essence of her remarks.

Pearse was evidently quite incapable of doing otherwise. By this point she even interpreted her own life through the prism of her deceased husband's theories. Shortly before his death he had begun to use the yolk sac surrounding vertebrate embryos as a key metaphor for an individuality impelled by the progressive differentiation of environment and organism. Not long afterwards Pearse began to write a biography of Scott Williamson, but seems to have realized that a conventional biographic approach would contradict his teachings. She wrote: "Dod's History can't be written without mine, mine affords the 'dark shutter' through which his 'light' can become differentiated, the 'printing' of the rhythm of its waves become apparent to the [...] eye." Scott Williamson became the growth medium for her own development, the prerequisite for her "specificity", the "eclection [sic] I gathered in the 'yolk sac' of the infancy of my maturing".[89]

Notes

1 Enid Mills, A Student in the Centre, 1948, WL, SA/PHC/B.5/21.
2 Ibid.
3 For a recent take on this issue, see: Lorrain Daston and Elizabeth Lunbeck, "Introduction. Observation Observed", in *Histories of Scientific Observation*, ed. Lorraine Daston and Elizabeth Lunbeck (Chicago, Ill.: University of Chicago Press, 2011), 1–9.
4 Pearse, *The Quality of Life*, 30 (original emphasis).
5 The Pioneer Health Centre, 1951, WL, SA/PHC/D.2/23/6, 2, 6.
6 Reminiscences of St Mary's Road Peckham, June/October 1984, WL, SA/PHC/C.20, 13.
7 Pearse, *The Quality of Life*, 91.
8 Michael Chance, "The Peckham Experiment: An Assessment", *Woman Health Officer* (August 1948).
9 Michael Chance, "Where from Peckham?", *The Lancet* (April 15, 1950): 727.
10 Ibid., 727.
11 Response to leader in *Medical Journal of Australia*, 1950, WL, SA/PHC/B.6/11.
12 M.L. Johnson, "Research in Social Organization. The Peckham Experiment", *Nature* 153 (1944): 269–270.
13 "Excursion into Utopia", *Medical Press* (September 19, 1945).

14 J.A. Ryle, "The Peckham Experiment", *Bulletin of Hygiene* (1944): 236.
15 I.H. Winner, "The End of the Peckham Experiment?", *Scientific Worker* 5, no. 4 (1950): 19–20.
16 This applies in particular to the work of Mike Savage. See for example *Identities and social change in Britain since 1940. The politics of method* (Oxford: Oxford University Press, 2010).
17 Mark Benney, "The Lost Chord," *International Women's News* (February 1944): 52–53.
18 David Stark Murray, "Doctors into Biologists", *Socialist Medical Association Bulletin* (September 1947).
19 Minutes, House Committee, August 20, 1949, WL, SA/PHC/A.1/6.
20 Donald Wilson to Pat Winsley, September 9, 1949, WL, SA/PHC/B.5/15. In his detailed analysis of the reasons for the closure of the centre, Philip Conford also cites the correspondence between Mary Langman and Douglas Trotter, which asserts that Major Short of the Health Trust regarded Scott Williamson as a megalomaniac, while Winfrey wanted to save the centre from its own directors: Conford, "Smashed by the National Health"?, 263.
21 Director's Report on the Centre, September 1949, WL, SA/PHC/A.1/6.
22 The team members were David V. Glass, demographer and former colleague of William Beveridge and Lancelot Hogben at LSE, J.N. Morris of the Social Medicine Research Unit of the Medical Research Council, M.L. Rosenheim, a doctor at University College Hospital, social psychologist John Rickman and Richard Scott of the Department of Public Health at the University of Edinburgh. See the covering letter by Major Short, November 1, 1949, BPS, Rickman Papers, P03/B/B/ 03–1.
23 According to the statement by Richard Scott, November 1949, BPS, Rickman Papers, P03/B/B/03–2, 4.
24 Minutes, General Purpose Committee, February 6, 1950, WL, SA/PHC/A.1/6.
25 Montagu to Winfrey, January 30, 1950, WL, SA/PHC/A.1/6.
26 See the correspondence at the WL, SA/PHC/B.5/16/1.
27 *The Times* (April 8, 1950).
28 The Passing of Peckham, 1951, WL, SA/PHC/B.6/13.
29 Conversely, it was scarcely fair of Pearse and Scott Williamson to accuse the new welfare regime of being uninterested in family health, an assessment that clashes with the medical authorities' broad concern for "problem families": Pat Starkey, "The Medical Officer of Health, the Social Worker, and the Problem Family, 1943 to 1968: The Case of Family Service Units", *Social History of Medicine* 11 (1998): 421–441.
30 Conford ("Smashed by the National Health"?, 264) speaks of "chemical triumphalism". This, he asserts, had begun to pervade food production as well. According to Conford this period was a generally difficult one for the quasi-ecological conception of a nutrient-rich environment so central to the PHC.
31 Dorothy Porter, "The decline of social medicine in Britain in the 1960s", in *Social medicine and medical sociology in the twentieth century*, ed. Dorothy Porter (Amsterdam: Rodopi, 1997), 97–119.
32 A.N. Rucker to J. Jackson, January 28, 1933, TNA, MH 52/159.
33 Montagu to Young, September 19, 1934, TNA, MH 52/159.
34 The Pioneer Health Centre at Peckham, September 24, 1934, TNA, MH 52/159, 5.
35 Donaldson, *Child of the Twenties*, 157.
36 Minutes, Board of Management/Management Committee, February 25, 1937, WL, SA/PHC/A.1/3.
37 Minutes, Executive Committee, March 21, 1939, WL, SA/PHC/A.1/4.
38 Untitled, May 2, 1939, WL, SA/PHC/B.3/15.
39 Annual Report 1938/39, WL, SA/PHC/A.2/11, 1, 3.

40 By 1943 at the latest the goal of evaluating the centre's economic aspects had been reinterpreted as a secondary feature of the research project and postponed. Pearse and Crocker, *The Peckham Experiment*, 320–322.

41 Mellanby to Hill, May 4, 1939, TNA, FD 1/299.

42 Hill to Mellanby, May 25, 1939, TNA, FD 1/299.

43 Scott Williamson to Hill, June 16, 1939, TNA, FD 1/299.

44 Previously the directors had also asked the National Council for Social Services and the Board of Education for help. A stalemate ensued: they were only prepared to provide funds if others did so too. Scott Williamson, meanwhile, repeatedly emphasized that he was less interested in financial support than in official recognition because this was likely to make private donors more willing to contribute (Scott Williamson to Herbert Sackville, June 19, 1939, TNA, ED 50/175). One of the PHC's main financial backers, Lord Nuffield, had in fact become sceptical: he made a donation of £5,000 dependent on a positive assessment by the Board of Education. He made good on his promise when the latter indicated its willingness to provide support (Nuffield to Sackville, June 12, 1939, TNA, ED 50/175). In June 1939 the crisis abated briefly when the Pilgrim Trust pledged £1,000 and the Halley Stewart Trust agreed to cover the researchers' salaries: Pilgrim Trust to Mellanby, July 31, 1939, TNA, ED 50/175.

45 The Passing of Peckham, 1951, WL, SA/PHC/B.6/13, 2.

46 Donaldson to Winfrey, March 16, 1945, WL, SA/PHC/B.4/5/2.

47 Memorandum on the Relation of the Peckham Health Centre to the National Health Act of 1948, undated [1948], WL, SA/PHC/B.5/16/2.

48 J.A. Charles to Mellanby, July 28, 1947, TNA, FD 1/299.

49 Mellanby to Charles, August 13, 1947, TNA, FD 1/299. An earlier attempt by Scott Williamson to sound out the MRC had got nowhere. Having supported research in social medicine before the war it had now begun to focus on clinical studies. Conford in fact ascribes some of the blame for the centre's demise to the MRC as a whole: Conford, "Smashed by the National Health?".

50 Minutes, Finance Committee and subcommittee, February 26, 1949, WL, SA/PHC/A.1/5.

51 Minutes, House Committee, December 6, 1949, WL, SA/PHC/A.1/6.

52 Minutes, House Committee, July 22, 1949, WL, SA/PHC/A.1/6.

53 Peckham Health Centre Renaming, undated, LMA, GLC/AR/HB/01.

54 The Passing of Peckham, 1951, WL, SA/PHC/B.6/13, 9.

55 Circular from Montagu, June 1951, gta, Giedion, 42-SG-36.

56 Peckham Health Centre – Allocation of Space for Conversion to Day-Nursery, General Practitioner and M. C.-Health Centre, undated [1951], LMA, LCC/PH/PHS/1/7.

57 Minutes, LCC Health Committee, undated [1950], WL, SA/PHC/B.6/4, 12.

58 Ibid., 17.

59 Press release, undated [1950], WL, SA/PHC/B.6/7.

60 "The End of an Experiment. Directors Give Reasons for Closing of the Peckham Health Centre", *The Manchester Guardian* (July 31, 1951).

61 Minutes, Sunday Meeting, undated [February 1950], WL, SA/PHC/B.6/2, 1, 7, 11.

62 "Health Centre as a show place. Ready for the 1951 Festival", *South London Observer* (August 17, 1950).

63 "Families say 'We'll march'", *Daily Herald* (April 6, 1950).

64 "Health Centre deputation sees eleven women M. P.s", *South London Press* (March 31, 1950).

65 Quoted in Stallibrass, *Being Me and Also Us*, 162.

66 As it happens, after the closure of the centre G.R. Boys, chair of the LCC's health committee, met with the members' association and showed great interest in "absorbing" them into the new centre: Pioneer Health Centre, PECKHAM. Use

of Premises, May 18, 1951, LMA, LCC/PH/PHS/1/7; "Health Centre: New Plan. Meeting the Criticisms", *South London Observer* (July 19, 1951). A compromise proposal was discussed in 1952 that would have involved the LCC renting out rooms for a self-administered "family club", at least on Saturday afternoons: Draft Rules of Family Club, undated [1952], LSE, COLL MISC 0521/2. The users, however, soon declared that they would not be taking part in any such club, as long as there was no plan to reinstate Pearse and Crocker: Peckham Members Association, March 1952, LSE, COLL MISC 0521/2.

67 Quoted in Stallibrass, *Being Me and Also Us*, 162–163.
68 "Doctors may fight this clinic", *South London Advertiser* (April 17, 1957).
69 See the documents in the LMA, LCC/CL/PH/1/133.
70 Huxley to Scott Williamson, June 30, 1950, WL, SA/PHC/B.6/6.
71 Huxley to Scott Williamson, July 19, 1950, WL, SA/PHC/D.1/7/17.
72 Mary Langman, Some notes on the implications of the Peckham experiment, June 1986, WL, SA/PHC/C.13, 2.
73 "George Scott Williamson", *The Lancet* (June 13, 1953): 1206–1207.
74 Financing PHC, undated [c. 1929], WL, SA/PHC/B.2/1, 2.
75 "The Basis of Planning. A Lecture given at the School of Planning and Research for National Development by Dr. Scott Williamson", *Architectural Association Journal* (November 1936): 182–186. See also Pearse and Crocker, *The Peckham Experiment*, 246.
76 Scott Williamson to Donaldson, June 7, 1950, WL, SA/PHC/B.6/10.
77 Scott Williamson to Winfrey, January 2, 1951, WL, SA/PHC/B.5/15.
78 Scott Williamson also identified himself with Einstein and Heisenberg. Scattered throughout his publications we find references to the insight that every measurement induces shifts in the state being measured. But Scott Williamson highlighted this not so much to critique deterministic thinking as to legitimize his own subjective method of observation: Chapter VIII, undated [early 1940s], WL, SA/PHC/D.2/9/3, 6.
79 Chapter I, WL, SA/PHC/D.2/9/3, 2.
80 Chapter VI, WL, SA/PHC/D.2/9/3, 3–4
81 Chapter VIII, WL, SA/PHC/D.2/9/3, 1, 7.
82 Chapter IX, WL, SA/PHC/D.2/9/3, 7.
83 Ibid., 12.
84 Mary Langman to Douglas Trotter, undated [1983], WL, SA/PHC/C.13.
85 Even Pearse had a hard time keeping track of her partner's neologisms: Alphabetical list of Scott Williamson's "terms", WL, SA/PHC/D.3/19.
86 Herbert Brewer, "Science, Synthesis and Sanity", *Eugenics Review* 58, no. 1 (1966): 33; Robert M. McGregor, "Living and Dying", *British Medical Journal* (January 29, 1966): 238.
87 Alex Comfort, "Comes the revolution", *New Scientist* (December 2, 1965).
88 "The Nature of Health", *The Expository Times* (August 1966): 335. Meanwhile, the book was well-received in esoteric circles, for instance in *The Aryan Path* 12 (1965). There had been a number of red flags. After reading an early manuscript in 1960, philosopher Henry Price, a man not averse to speculative thought, had written that the text achieved the minimum requirement for clarity – but only just, he seems to imply. But Price considered Scott Williamson's Latin barbaric: "tactic" is not derived from "tangere", he has no idea what an "inventurer" is, and "mutation" has little to do with "mutual". Price to Donaldson, May 27, 1960, WL, SA/PHC/D.4/24.
89 Dod's biography can't be written without mine, August 7, 1956, WL, SA/PHC/E.4.

11 "Peckham" after the Pioneer Health Centre and the changing discourse of health (1959–)

Those who abandon the realm of the measurable, as George Scott Williamson and Innes Pearse did in the early 1940s, risk ending up in the sphere of religion. To begin the history of the impact of the Peckham Experiment with a leap forward in time: the most recent work penned by a former Peckham staff member is theological in nature. Douglas Trotter's 2003 book *Wholeness and Holiness* goes into very little depth about the history of the PHC. It does, however, demonstrate that it is possible to forge links between Scott Williamson's holism and the exegesis of the early Christian theologians, as well as New Age ideas such as James Lovelock's "Gaia hypothesis".[1]

Trotter's publication is the latest in a long line of attempts by centre staff to develop and disseminate the insights gleaned there. The first to achieve success was Alison Stallibrass, who attempted to draw out the centre's lessons for pedagogy. By 1952 she had founded a so-called "free-choice-playgroup" and in the early 1970s she published several texts on her experiences with it, making connections with contemporary debates on anti-authoritarian and holistic education. In 1974, in her book *The Self-Respecting Child*, she asserted that the main goal of all education was "becoming oneself".[2] With the help of numerous examples from the centre she described pedagogical methods intended to prevent the self-alienation she found to be prevalent in modern society. Above all Stallibrass recommended that small children be given the opportunity to test out their own locomotor skills autonomously, through improvised seesaws, slides and climbing frames. In connection with this she provided tips on non-intervention for educators. The core message was that children themselves are the best judges of their own limits and abilities.

At the same time other former members of centre staff were taking concrete steps to establish a new iteration of the institution. In 1967 Aubrey Collings, a businessman who had worked at the centre as a student and had even lived briefly with Pearse and Scott Williamson,[3] began to collect money for a "Peckham"-like health centre in Stockton on Tees in the north of England, the so-called Thornaby Project. He made approaches to centre veterans – who had by this point established a Peckham Committee – and the architect of the old building, Owen Williams, who expressed interest in designing a new one.[4] The project, however, rapidly petered out when the committee fell out with Collings. The main bone of contention was the latter's unwillingness to cling dogmatically to the template of the old centre. The Peckham Committee was particularly opposed to his idea of providing medical treatment in the centre. In a lengthy letter Collings underlined that to create the kind of health-promoting environment the committee envisaged was in itself a form of therapy. There were, he went on, simply too many "strings attached" for a cooperative venture with former PHC staff.[5] The fact that the MRC and Ministry of Health roundly rejected his proposal may have added to his disappointment.[6] Apparently these institutions remembered only too well the problems associated with the closed centre.

The committee, however, gained new supporters. In 1970 it planned to establish a centre in Somers Town in the London borough of Camden, based on the thesis of architecture student Peter Ray, who basically gave Williams's building a futuristic update. This building project, which would evidently have required the demolition of several blocks of terraced housing,[7] also fizzled out quickly. Nonetheless, the committee was soon able to make use of Ray's blueprints when it began to draw up plans for a health centre in the new town of Glenrothes in Scotland. Pearse, Trotter and Langman worked on this project for more than ten years.[8] Having learned from past experience, they strove to forge links with existing institutions, seeking cooperation with the nearby University of St Andrews. They even approached the World Health Organization (WHO) in Copenhagen.[9] In 1979 they almost managed to acquire a plot of land but the plan came to grief due to lack of funds. Tellingly, at their meetings the members of the committee had repeatedly put off clarifying the exact nature of the project's objectives.[10]

(Post-)modernization

A certain inability on the part of the committee members to revise their plans, which hampered efforts to create a new centre, can probably be put down to Pearse's influence:[11] at this point in time, in the shape of *The Quality of Life*, she was trying to perpetuate her own version of her husband's intellectual legacy. Just a few years after her death in 1978 – she made over her entire estate to the Peckham Committee[12] – the Peckham Experiment then underwent a minor renaissance in the discourse of social and health policy.[13] This was partly the result of a publishing offensive in the early 1980s, preceded by the initial attempts at historicization mentioned earlier – the latter explain the ample documentary record on the centre. Various individuals amalgamated archival documents and carried out interviews in order to obtain material for texts that, now, increasingly highlighted the centre's focus on personal freedom. In 1988 Kenneth Barlow, who had worked there as a doctor after the war, published the book *Recognising Health*, which radically modernized his former superiors' vocabulary – the new key terms were "system" and "participation". Nonetheless Barlow was unable to cast off outmoded views entirely. In a polemical vein he wrote that while there was a lot of talk nowadays of single-parent families, from a biological point of view it was all "nonsense".[14]

Community physician Alex Scott-Samuel, meanwhile, was more focused on forging new connections. In the mid 1980s he had initiated meetings between a group of younger health experts and former centre staff members and users. These gave rise to the PHC Project Team, predecessor to the Pioneer Health Foundation, which is still active today. In 1989 Scott-Samuel published the essay *Total Participation, Total Health*, in which he underlined that the Peckham Experiment had been decades ahead of its time. It had pre-empted the now omnipresent demand – within the framework of "holistic health care" – to consider not just the sick organ but the entire human being and the risks to which he is exposed. Unlike Barlow, Scott-Samuel identified concrete points of contact with existing institutions, namely patients' and neighbourhood initiatives, self-help groups and so-called look-after-yourself courses. One post-modern buzzword appears here for the first time. The Peckham Experiment, Scott-Samuel contends, had shown that "social networks" must be taken into account when it comes to issues of health. It had thus anticipated the "shift from a medical to a social model of health". Scott-Samuel was also more comfortable with "alternative" lifestyles, constructing a version of the experiment adapted to the pluralist ethos typical of many social movements in the 1980s. While the concept of the family had changed since the 1930s, he pointed out, "human needs and potentialities" were unchanging.[15]

The Peckham advocates' publications were well received; they made a snug fit with the political debates of the time. Many critics claimed that the National Health Service Reorganisation Act of 1973 had made the NHS even more labyrinthine, even though the reorganization itself was a response to pressure from newly established patients' initiatives and other interest groups, which were calling for greater citizen participation.[16] In 1974 a small number of (rather unsuccessful) so-called community health councils were established and more funds were made available for follow-up studies on patient satisfaction. Three years later a government White Paper, *Prevention and Health*, recommended a social policy more focused on individual needs, while also calling for greater personal responsibility. When Margaret Thatcher took office the government built on this, stepping up state health promotion efforts in a campaign that made significant use of the advertising industry.[17] We can thus discern a direct connection between the efforts made by the heirs to the centre and the political climate of the late 1970s and 1980s. Interesting in this context is the fact that Barlow put the NHS's tremendous financial losses partly down to its failure to sufficiently incentivize people to work on their own health.[18] Stallibrass's, Barlow's and Scott-Samuel's publications thus contributed to a debate that formed the background to the reforms announced by Thatcher in 1988; these provided for part-privatization, that is, competition between the suppliers of medical services. It would be very unfair, however, to identify the same neoliberal spirit at work in the above authors' writings. In particular, Scott-Samuel's ideas on neighbourhood medical care were inspired by the critique of institutional medicine as anonymizing and incapacitating, which was articulated by widely read authors such as Ivan Illich at the time. But this did not prevent the Thatcher government from adroitly co-opting such critiques in another White Paper entitled *Working for Patients*, published in 1989.[19]

As it happens, in the second half of the twentieth century the advantages of local health centres were discussed beyond liberal political contexts, broadly understood. As indicated above, the National Health Service Act of 1946 had provided for comprehensive health care for the British population through health centres. This project, however, failed due to resistance from the medical lobby, lack of funds and the way responsibilities were organized within the NHS – to the great disappointment of the left-wing opponents of the PHC, in the SMA for example, whose supporters had hoped for a more decentralized system with greater citizen participation, and were soon criticizing the NHS, much like the Peckham directors, as a "national sickness service".[20] Initially, funding for the NHS had in fact flowed mainly into the construction of hospitals. Health centres were built only within the framework of new housing estates; by 1960 there were just ten in total in England and Wales.[21] Still, after 1966 a number of so-called primary care centres or primary health area centres were established, which provided dental care and advisory services and served as clearing houses for hospitals. A few years later health centres also became a hot topic internationally, for example at the WHO, which advocated them primarily as an apt means of improving medical care in the "developing countries".[22] At the same time the governments of Canada and Finland planned networks of health centres, with tribute being paid time and again to the PHC's pioneering role.[23] Little, however, was made of its "biological" insights. Again, the centre provided even supporters of the expansion of the welfare state with key terms. It symbolized the location-independent production of equal living conditions, a crucial source of legitimacy for the state spending expanding so dramatically in the 1960s. It was not until the late 1980s that the principles of decentralization, participation in decision-making and a market orientation then began to overlap.[24]

From social engineer to social entrepreneur

We have now come full circle and find ourselves returning to the 2007 debate in the *Guardian* mentioned in the introduction. The first key issue here was to what extent the centre could contribute to constructive arguments on participation and citizen empowerment within the health care system. The second related to the privatization and the commodification of medical care. During the general election campaign of 1997, under the leadership of Tony Blair, New Labour had promised to abolish the "internal market", which Conservative governments had previously begun to establish within the NHS. Blair, however, continued the programme during his second term in office. The UK now saw the development of an increasing number of semi-private social welfare institutions, about whose efficacy and political implications opinions differ sharply. The best examples are the so-called healthy living centres that have appeared in many major British cities, often funded by the National Lottery. They are supposed to create incentives for those on low incomes to take up sports in order to lower the long-term costs of the welfare state. Incidentally, for a number of years the district of Peckham itself has been home to the much-praised Peckham Pulse Centre, a municipal swimming pool with adjoining fitness studio, which are subsidized by Southwark Council.

The template for the healthy living centres was the Bromley by Bow Centre in East London, which is worth taking a closer look at: until recently the Pioneer Health Foundation highlighted it as exemplary on its website.[25] But the centre in Bromley is also interesting because here a charismatic autocrat played a role that may seem rather familiar. In the mid 1980s Andrew Mawson took up the role of pastor for the United Reformed Church in Bromley by Bow, East London, an area with a large number of immigrants and high unemployment. Mawson resolved to completely revamp his poorly attended church, including its architecture. It was transformed into a blend of community, information and business centre, with a health centre being added in 1997. To this day the Bromley centre provides medical advice, language courses and motivational training, but its main focus is on fostering business enterprises. For example, the staff help locals establish and run micro-enterprises such as groceries, in part by providing loans, with the interest being reinvested in the centre. Thus, the Bromley by Bow Centre seems a bit like a revenant of the settlement houses of the late nineteenth century in the East End of London, not excepting its ideology: for Mawson makes no bones about the fact that for him state social policy causes rather than resolves many of the problems experienced by the residents of Bromley. Social policy specialists and welfare agencies, he contends, know nothing about the specific circumstances of those on benefits, which thus fail to make any real impact. Furthermore Mawson takes a swipe at what he regards as the muddled notions of justice expounded by many in the Labour Party and assails its supposedly weak leadership. More importantly, there is no overlooking the similarity between his views and the quasi-anthropological arguments put forward by the centre's directors more than 50 years earlier. Mawson, for example, who has at least once publicly invoked Pearse and Scott Williamson,[26] writes:

> We know that every human being has a unique talent. By applying these talents in local communities it is possible to make them strong and vibrant instead of soulless and "deprived". Health is not just about clinical solutions but also about the links with wider social networks.[27]

Mawson stylizes himself as a man of action, a down-to-earth social entrepreneur rather than an expertocratic social *engineer*, as evident in his ambiguously entitled book *Making Communities Work*.[28] He has been ennobled, sits in the House of Lords as a crossbencher and prides himself on having advised Prime Ministers Blair and Cameron and having been courted by Gordon Brown. Mawson has since completed the metamorphosis from pastor to businessman. He now runs an agency that promises to optimize the new social institutions established since the late 1990s in the wake of the privatization of state services, such as youth centres.

As with the Peckham Experiment, in no way do I dismiss the improvements in people's lives brought about by the centre in Bromley. But Mawson's self-stylization as a one-man alternative to the welfare state is problematic. It fits only too well with a practice that has been described as governing through community. This refers to a form of local micromanagement that encourages the disadvantaged to embrace an actively entrepreneurial identity as an ethical imperative.[29] For many advocates of this approach the aim is to abolish the scattergun of the welfare state in favour of non-profit initiatives, run along strictly economic lines, which can respond nimbly to shifts in the labour market.

Notes

1 Trotter, J. Douglas, *Wholeness and Holiness. A Study in Human Ethology and the Holy Trinity* (Glasgow: Pioneer Health Foundation, 2003).
2 Stallibrass, *The Self-Respecting Child*, 180.
3 He described this as an enlightening experience: Aubrey Collings, The Thornaby Project, January 29, 1968, WL, SA/PHC/C.3.
4 Williams to Allan Pepper, December 7, 1967, WL, SA/PHC/C.3.
5 Collings to the PHC-Committee, June 8, 1969, WL, SA/PHC/C.3.
6 Mary Langman to Collings, June 24, 1968, WL, SA/PHC/C.3.
7 Peter Ray, Comprehensive Design Project: Final Design Thesis, Part Two of the Examination in Architecture, June 1970, WL, SA/PHC/C.4/1.
8 Notes providing a context for the PHC Ltd., archive papers relating to project proposals after the 1950 closure, March 1998, WL, SA/PHC/C.2. Meanwhile Jack Donaldson, a member of the House of Lords since 1967, sought to keep memories of the PHC alive by mentioning it in many of his contributions: *Hansard* 287 (1967): 1518–1519.
9 Minutes of a meeting with WHO representatives, October 2, 1977, WL, SA/PHC/C.10.
10 Minutes, Health Science Committee, February 19, 1980, WL, SA/PHC/C.14/2.
11 Report on the Research Situation of the Pioneer Health Centre by IHP, June 1978, WL, SA/PHC/C.11.
12 Minutes, executive committee, Pioneer Health Centre Ltd., March 26, 1979, WL, SA/PHC/C.14/1.
13 Jane Lewis and Barbara Brookes. "A reassessment of the work of the Peckham Health Centre, 1926–1951", *Health and Society* 61 (1983): 307–350; Donald C. Ramsom, "Random notes: The legacy of the Peckham experiment", *Family Systems Medicine* 10 (1983): 104–108.; D.F. Duncan, "The Peckham experiment: a pioneering exploration of wellness", *Health Values* 9 (1985): 40–43; Kenneth Barlow, "The Peckham Experiment", *Medical History* 29 (1985): 264–271; Joel Elkes, "Past/Future Conjoined: Note from the USA on the Present Edition", *Social Medicine* 4 (2009 [1985]): 192–194; Stephen King Hall, "45 years ago – the Pioneer Health Centre, Peckham", *Journal of the Royal Society of Medicine* 82

(1989): 577–578; John Pemberton, "The Peckham-Experiment", *Journal of Public Health Policy* 12 (1991): 542–544.

14 Kenneth Barlow, *Recognising Health* ([London:] McCarrison Society, 1988), 88.
15 Scott-Samuel, *Total Participation, Total Health*, 25, 30–31, 28, 10, 13
16 Glen O'Hara, "The Complexities of 'Consumerism': Choice, Collectivism and Participation within Britain's National Health Service, c. 1961–c. 1979", *Social History of Medicine* 25 (2013): 288–304.
17 Virginia Berridge, *Health and Society in Britain since 1939* (New York: Cambridge University Press, 1999), 87–91.
18 Barlow, *Recognising health*, 131.
19 Alex Mold, "Making the Patient-Consumer in Margaret Thatcher's Britain", *The Historical Journal* 54 (2011): 509–528.
20 Stewart, *The Political Economy of the British National Health Service*, 453.
21 Lewis and Brookes, "The Peckham Health Centre", 158.
22 Roemer, *Evaluation of Community Health Centres*, 17.
23 For example: *The Community Health Centre in Canada. Report of the Community Health Centre Project to the Health Ministers* (Ottawa: Information Canada, 1972/73). Peckham is mentioned in vol. 3, 2–4.
24 This overlap is evident in the debates within the sub-organizations of the WHO: *The Role of Health Centres in the Development of Urban Health Systems. Report of a WHO Study Group on primary Health Care in Urban Areas* (Geneva: World Health Organization, 1992); and Robert Kohn, *The health centre concept in primary health care* ([Geneva:] World Health Organization, 1983), 10. The PHC Project Team also got involved at the margins: see for example The Peckham Experiment and the Healthy City, WHO Symposium Zagreb, September 1988, WL, SA/PHC/C.19/5; Self Sustaining Human Ecology: A paper for the WHO Healthy Cities Symposium, Stockholm 1990, WL, SA/PHC/C.19/7; and Managing Change, Healthy Cities Symposium, Barcelona, Spain, September 25–29, 1991, WL, SA/PHC/C.19/8.
25 http://thephf.org/index.php/relevance-today (accessed July 8, 2013).
26 "Reorganisation of the NHS," http://amawsonpartnerships.com/lords/reorganisation-of-the-nhs/ (accessed December 17, 2017).
27 "Story", http://amawsonpartnerships.com/story/ (accessed July 8, 2013).
28 Andrew Mawson, *The Social Entrepreneur. Making Communities Work* (London: Atlantic, 2008). It should be noted that the term "social entrepreneur" was popularized in the mid-1990s by Michael Young, well known as one of the authors of the influential sociological study *Family and Kinship in East London* (1957), which explored the effects of the post-war building programme on the traditional working-class milieu. Young is also considered to be one of the key sources of inspiration for New Labour. More importantly, in the 1940s, as member of the PEP Health Group, he was involved in the development of the NHS and in the early 1960s he helped kick off the first debates on consumer rights and patient participation. In 1984 (in *Self Health* magazine) Young too recalled the PHC; it was, he asserted, a source of ideas on how to improve the "National Disease Service": Michael Young, "The Peckham Experiment", *Self Health* 10 (1984): 11.
29 Rose, *Powers of Freedom*.

12 Preliminary conclusion
The Pioneer Health Centre as liberal missing link?

We have arrived in the present, a good time to take stock of the institutional history of the centre and its successors. From the vantage point of its main interpreters, Pearse and Scott Williamson, this history presents a mixed picture: during the centre's existence they witnessed a rapid shift in the degree of attention paid to their project and ideas. The parameters of non-state welfare initiatives in the United Kingdom changed quickly in the middle decades of the twentieth century. Partly as a consequence of their attempts to influence these dynamics, Pearse and Scott Williamson were caught in their wake. Within just a few years the Peckham Experiment was wrenched from a state of relative obscurity into the media spotlight – in the late 1940s the experiment's directors even found themselves at the UN General Assembly, the symbolic centre of global politics. Not long afterwards, however, their project was on the rocks. It was arguably a failure. Pearse and Scott Williamson had clearly become isolated even within the scientific community.

In the late 1930s the centre had stood at the intersection of debates on nature and society, social medicine and social policy, the country's future, personal development, state intervention and local administration. But in the following decade most commentators in science, politics and the press, while viewing the centre as a source of stimulation, by no means considered it unconditionally worthy of emulation. One of the reasons for this was that the centre turned out to be an economic disappointment. Initial hopes that it might demonstrate that a healthy population, in both the narrower and broader senses of the term, need cost society virtually nothing and could be achieved with little administrative effort, proved illusory. Partly due to their inability or unwillingness to admit this (even to themselves), the two directors had shifted focus away from social policy towards a quasi-anthropological biology. But they made excessive claims in light of their findings, and fatally, they did so at a point in time when techniques for establishing scientific evidence had begun to change, with a marked shift towards a "hard" form of statistical data analysis. Paradoxically, this discrepancy gave rise to argumentational ambiguities that may have kept alive interdisciplinary interest in the centre over the medium term, as we will see in a moment. In the first instance, though, its main effect was to irritate the project's financial supporters, prompting them to back off. For many years this incongruity also hampered efforts to revive the project in a new form.

If we include the centre's members in our appraisal we might well consider them among its beneficiaries. They had a fairly affordable leisure centre at their disposal thanks to the financial subsidies provided by the centre's supporters. Furthermore, if we are to believe the medical data from the centre, the members' resistance to illness had increased appreciably. But ironically, this did not verify the scientists' theories. One might in fact assert that the members' improved health exemplified the positive effects of the very form of material redistribution to which the centre sought to provide an alternative. The social situation in "Peckham", however, was more multifaceted than a neat identification of winners and losers conveys. This is evident in the complex ruptures arising from the way in which day-to-day life at the centre was interpreted. As indicated earlier, many visitors entered the building on St Mary's Road with expectations moulded by their reading of publications on the project. They encountered a centre that was quite ready for them: in the post-war era, many users of the centre were clearly prepared to affirm the picture the researchers had painted of them. There is no need to assume they were motivated by self-interest. Partly out of a sense of responsibility and genuine interest in Scott Williamson's and Pearse's theories, a number of members appear to have more or less consciously orchestrated scenes of natural self-optimization and mutual stimulation as described by the scientists. An overall appraisal of the centre would thus also require us to include rather hazy variables: feelings, moods and personal experiences of success. There is some evidence that for most of its users the centre was a special and especially harmonious place; it appears that many of them perceived the staff as interesting, unusually approachable representatives of another class with a genuine concern for their well-being.

However we view "Peckham", then, we never end up with a coherent whole – because it never was one. So what is it that makes the study of the Pioneer Health Centre (along with its failure and its former staff members' attempts to revive it) more than just part of the history of a London neighbourhood? What can this history do for us other than demonstrate how the protagonists marginalized themselves? What does it tell us about the shifting societal contexts that engendered this marginalization? Here we must return to the Foucauldian ideas on twentieth-century "regimes of activation" mentioned in the introduction. From a highly elevated vantage point we might regard the centre as an example of "biopolitics" as such. It would then appear as a variant of a mode of governance that aims to lure out life itself and render it productive. In this connection we might use the centre to study how the application of power shifted away from deviation to the average, away from "problem" groups to the majority population. This analysis, however, does little more than confirm a highly formulaic grand theory.

Focusing specifically on the British history of the nineteenth and twentieth centuries, we might also conclude that "Peckham" forms a missing link that has persisted across historical eras between (economically) liberal ideologies, one disguised, as it were, as scientistic (and architectural) reformism. There is certainly an affinity between the ideas about the human being underlying the self-help practices that sprang up in the second half of the nineteenth century, those central to the mid-century "biological" reasoning at the centre and those inherent in the neoliberal turn in the early 1980s. This is particularly apparent when we consider that the new notion of marketization as a remedy for societal ills was extolled – with the aid of a deft populism – as the restoration of Victorian values.[1] We might question such claims of continuity, however, by pointing out that in the wartime and post-war UK even the exponents of state intervention expressed concern about robbing people of their initiative and self-determination through an excess of welfare and benefits.[2] In any case, the simplifying distinction between the advocates of egalitarianism, dirigisme and centralism on the one hand and a market orientation, personal responsibility and individual performance on the other has a history of its own. Since the 1970s this distinction has been deployed whenever the welfare state is blamed for the UK's alleged loss of a culture of competition. This supposed loss is in turn frequently identified as the mental cause of the British economy's structural weakness – if not as a key element in the decline of a formerly dominant global empire over the course of the twentieth century.[3] But those who describe the solidarity-based national community with its post-war consensus as a lost paradise – in view of the frigid social atmosphere generated by the alleged new paradigm ("no such thing as society") – are also simplifying things.

The interpretation-generator of "Peckham" is undoubtedly still active. And as we get nearer to the present, neoliberal ideas do in fact occupy an ever-greater share of the interpretive landscape. This is apparent in social entrepreneur Mawson's reference to the experiment. It would, however, be wrong to impute to the centre a secret *political* agenda or to stylize it as a systematically designed test bed for governmental practices consonant with the much-vaunted "new spirit of capitalism",[4] as some of the architectural historians mentioned in the introduction would have it. For this would be to ignore the fact that one of the consequences of Pearse and Scott Williamson's biologism, with its critique of modern civilization, was their lack of belief in politics, especially in the sense of institutionalized antagonism. After all, their self-manoeuvring into the discursive margins in the late 1940s had much to do with their refusal to participate in the political process. Certainly, the centre directors acted opportunistically in some instances. But when it came to their grand theories they were imperturbable. From a present-day perspective this does not necessarily make them any more appealing. As late as the 1970s Pearse and some of her colleagues articulated a world view that conceptualized same-sex love, life as a single person and blended families as unnatural, degenerate phenomena. Their style of thought has little in common with the tolerance of – or rather indifference towards – different lifestyles that now tends to characterize even the most economically liberal political beliefs. And it is quite out of synch with consumer markets that discern the potential for commodification in the most minor of lifestyle differences.

At most indirectly – in light of a notion of personal aptitudes whose development could be hampered by flawed societal institutions – can we discern a certain affinity with the meritocratic thinking of the post-war era.[5] It thus seems unhelpful to think of the significance of the Peckham Experiment in terms of continuities in political ideology. We can, however, recognize its legacy in the subliminal persistence of specific elements of the scientific knowledge it generated, despite all the contemporary criticisms made of the research practices at the Pioneer Health Centre. At times, the ways in which Pearse, Crocker and Scott Williamson sought to conceptualize their experiences at the centre, the combination of metaphors on which they drew, are a hair's breadth away from outright nonsense. Yet their very polysemy has enabled others to use the "Peckham" directors' statements like a construction kit. In the final chapter I thus seek to demonstrate that since the 1940s their publications have left behind clear traces in the knowledge stocks cultivated by three societal subsystems. It is chiefly *anarchists* and *architects* and, more important still, *social psychologists* who have taken inspiration from the experiment. In analysing these recipients I will of necessity distance myself from the centre at times as I seek, on a modest scale, to cast new light on the history of knowledge in the second half of the twentieth century. It is important to keep in mind here that what applies to the transfer of concepts between countries or scientific cultures applies even more to rediscoveries: such time travel entails the loss of certain meanings, which are superseded by others. But these new elements tell us a great deal about the era in question.

Notes

1 Florence Sutcliffe-Braithwaite, "Neo-Liberalism and Morality in the Making of Thatcherite Social Policy", *The Historical Journal 55* (2012): 497–520.
2 Abigail Beach, "Forging a 'nation of participants'. Political and Economic Planning in Labour's Britain", in *The Right to Belong. Citizenship and National Identity in Britain, 1930–1960*, eds Abigail Beach and Richard Weight (London: I. B. Tauris, 1998), 98–115; and Pat Thane, "The 'Big Society' and the 'Big State': Creative Tension or Crowding Out?", *Twentieth Century British History* 23 (2012): 408–429. Conversely, in its early days – that is, contemporaneous with the Peckham Experiment – even pioneers of neoliberalism like the Mont Pèlerin Society (founded in 1947) did not reject every form of state interventionism *per se*. Ben Jackson, "The Origins of Neo-Liberalism: the Free Economy and the Strong State, 1930–1947", *The Historical Journal* 53 (2010): 129–151.
3 Jim Tomlinson, "Thrice Denied: 'Declinism' as a Recurrent Theme in British History in the Long Twentieth Century", *Twentieth Century British History* 20 (2009): 227–251.
4 Luc Boltanski and Ève Chiapello, *The New Spirit of Capitalism* (London/New York: Verso, 2005).
5 On the continuities between the eugenic theories of the 1930s and post-war meritocratic thinking, see Chris Renwick, *British sociology's lost biological roots: a history of futures past* (Basingstoke: Palgrave Macmillan, 2012).

13 The promise of Peckham
Hidden legacies

Anarchist appropriations

The fears expressed by socialist critics of the centre were misplaced. It was not conservative opinion leaders who regarded the Peckham Experiment as a source of scientific support for their views; as indicated earlier it was chiefly anarchists who selectively cultivated its memory. Representatives of the London Anarchist Group, including journalist Herbert Read, had become aware of the experiment before the war was over. In his 1943 review of *The Peckham Experiment*, Read too interpreted the centre primarily as a sociological research project. As such, he contended, it had shown that the absence of a strict external order was particularly likely to facilitate the emergence of competent social communities.[1] The same year Read wrote to journalist Louise Morgan regarding the centre: "I had shared the common impression that it was an up-to-date clinic of some sort, and I never had the slightest suspicion that a social experiment so nearly touching my own ideals was taking place almost under my eyes." He had long hoped for scientific corroboration of his political views and would forever be in Scott Williamson's debt: "The first person I shall talk to about it is Karl Mannheim, and I expect that he will be very sorry that he has not had the privilege of including the volume [*The Peckham Experiment*] in the Library of Sociology."[2]

In 1944 Read asked Scott Williamson to contribute to a special issue of *World Review*. Here, among other contributors, Mannheim and Anna Freud attempted to answer the question: "What conditions are necessary for the development of man and society to a high degree of potentiality?"[3] Read's own contribution consisted of ruminations on the "biological vitality of the community as such", to which, he claimed, "plans for social betterment" had so far paid meagre attention. He expressed scepticism about mass democracy, evoking a romanticized image of the Middle Ages. The main problem of the present era, he averred, was widespread social apathy. The crucial step towards overcoming it was to answer the "question of social size", particularly with respect to the (excessive) scope of state power. Only science, according to Read, could provide this answer.[4]

We can hardly fail to note the overlap with Scott Williamson's views. His contribution, however, went unpublished. Scott Williamson had essentially ignored Read's guidelines. Instead he had submitted a short text on the difference between technicians and scientists, one featuring his usual word games ("plant" rather than "plan" should be the name of the game), and pervaded by multiple barely comprehensible neologisms.[5] Nonetheless, the London anarchists continued to study the centre, particularly after its reopening. In 1947 John Hewetson, himself a physician and co-editor of what was then the leading organ of British anarchism, *Freedom*, published an enthusiastic account of his visit to Peckham: "On coming to the Centre, one feels that a world of frustration and chaos has been left behind. One is amongst people who are understanding the benefits of responsibility, initiative, self-respect and are fast learning the art of living." Hewetson seems almost relieved: "[I]f the premises on which the Peckham Centre is founded [are found] to be correct, then not only will they be a vindication of Dr. Scott Williamson's theories but of the sound biological bases of the Anarchist philosophy."[6] Scott Williamson was aware of the anarchists' veneration. He accepted invitations to speak before the Anarchist Group on Tavistock Square on a number of occasions.[7] In 1951, however, he sent a furious retort to the *Medical Press* when it described him as an anarchist: "I am not an anarchist nor do I believe in anarchy – not even in the Kropotkin type. I do not find anarchy in Nature. Nature obeys her own laws as the physicists have demonstrated." Yet he added:

> On the other hand, equally I do not believe in "Leaders", not even in those persons who have acquired diplomas in leadership. [...] Leadership is, in fact, no respector [sic] of persons and seems to be a function of the environment, that is to say, it appears to grow out of circumstances. [...] The foolish concept that Autonomy results in Anarchy has, I think, been completely disproved by what happened in Peckham, where Autonomy resolved itself into Autarchy – self government through self discipline.[8]

In light of such statements it comes as no surprise that 15 years later, in the aforementioned special issue of *Anarchy*, Hewetson's successor Colin Ward was full of praise for Scott Williamson's experiment. In 1966 he put it on the same level as the insights of Bakunin and Proudhon.[9] Ward had visited the centre himself in 1949; for the rest of his life he never tired of expressing his enthusiasm about it.[10] Notably, Ward worked as an architect for many years and was to become an important supporter of the British squatting movement. His interest in the Peckham Experiment is thus not only representative of anarchists' appropriations of the centre myth but also sheds light on why it made such a splash in the discourse of architecture. What is more, as I will demonstrate in a moment, Ward's views are a striking example of the shift in the interpretation of the experiment evident in other contexts of reception as well.

The Peckham Experiment as seen by city planners and architects

Shortly after it was opened Owen Williams's glass construction became a hot topic in transnational architectural circles. In 1935 former Bauhaus director Walter Gropius, who had recently emigrated to England, praised the building as the only interesting one in the country.[11] Two years later it entered the canon of modernism, appearing in the catalogue of the *Modern Architecture in England* exhibition, previously held at the New York Museum of Modern Art.[12] Overall the building played a significant role in the renewal of British architecture in the late 1930s. Students of the Architectural Association School of Architecture, including many influential post-war planners, were enthusiastic about Williams's rationalistic building, but also about the research project being pursued within it.[13] In 1936 Scott Williamson was invited to give a lecture at the AA School, where he took the opportunity to warn of the dangers of planning euphoria. His experiment, he contended, made it plain that the individual must be considered against the "overwhelming background" of his environment. His research was in the process of revealing ways of tapping the individual's "potentiality, its latent capacity for development, [of facilitating] its maximum fruition". Buildings, he explained, could be an obstacle to this process. Architects ought to give them expiry dates if they were not to eventually degenerate into prisons.[14]

The PHC also cropped up in the city planning debate of the early 1940s. Here it was generally linked with a much-discussed new approach to urban planning centred on the so-called neighbourhood unit. The idea was to provide housing estates and urban districts earmarked for "redevelopment" with a clear sociospatial structure.[15] Urban agglomerations were to be kept separate, limited in size and oriented towards a community centre. The latter would serve as a place for neighbours to meet and simultaneously as a locus for social institutions, educational establishments and shops. This, it was hoped, would make it easier for highly integrated communities to emerge. First propagated in the United States in 1924, the concept of the neighbourhood enjoyed a particularly enthusiastic reception in Britain. By creating spaces on a "human scale" its exponents hoped to establish the kind of close neighbourly relations that seemed to have become a rarity in the modern city. We can thus regard the neighbourhood unit as the counterpart of some of the ideas put forward by the Peckham directors in that it was in practice an attempt to ascertain the ideal spatial extent of residential areas. Here architects often deployed the same anthropometric category the Peckham researchers sometimes claimed to have used to measure the centre's catchment area: walking distance.[16]

More than anyone else it was architect Jacqueline Tyrwhitt, research director at the School of Planning and Regional Reconstruction in London, who brought the project in Peckham to the attention of influential urban planners.[17] She arranged for Scott Williamson to be invited to the CIAM (Congrès Internationaux d'Architecture Moderne) conference of 1951 in

Hoddesdon, Hertfordshire, briefly making him the idol of this avant-garde organization.[18] Around this time the CIAM too was beginning to address "soft" anthropological and social psychological aspects of city planning. The organization backed off a little from the paradigm of strict functional division embodied in the famous (or notorious) "Athens Charter" formulated after its 1933 conference: its members increasingly discussed ways of creating spatial settings conducive to processes of social integration. Scott Williamson's speech thus fit neatly with the organizers' views. He underlined that while human potential was biologically determined, it was possible to expedite its realization. The key requirement here was to provide people with an environment that gave them as many options as possible: "The power of the architect to fix the conditions in which life and living has to take place, is tremendous – almost frightening."[19] But Scott Williamson made it clear that this power was by no means inevitably destructive: prior to the establishment of the centre, the residents of Peckham had been in an embryonic state, "incapable of exercising their will". They had now fully matured and had formed a community entirely by themselves.

The modernists' interest in unleashing human potential, however, entailed certain risks for them. At the ninth CIAM conference in Aix-en-Provence, just two years after Scott Williamson's lecture, a group of younger architects sceptical of established functionalist ideas, Team 10, highlighted the advantages of the much-maligned big-city slums: in social terms they seemed far livelier than the experts' planned housing schemes. Remarkably, even these critics of the avant-gardists – who were increasingly denounced as authoritarian – referred to the PHC. They viewed it as an antidote to the older generation's obsession with order.

The publishing history of a sketch of the centre building (Figure 13.1), reproduced in the official 1951 conference report, may give us some idea of the factors facilitating this reinterpretation. Interestingly, this drawing does not show the centre's architecture.[20] Instead it visualizes a number of activities that took place inside a transparent structure liberated from its facade. Here everything seems to be in a state of flux: the schematic figures and the outlines of the furnishings overlap, the walls are permeable, the inside and outside of the building distinguished merely by broken lines. We may interpret this graphic dissolving of boundaries in various ways. The X-ray-like perspective might suggest a near-omnipotent penetration of what is portrayed. But it might also represent what Scott Williamson and his colleagues had begun to call the holistic, "bioscopic" perspective: ultimately, the viewer also sees the researchers at work in their laboratories and offices on the first floor. The objective observer's standpoint, disconnected from what is happening, has swept away the normativity of the experts' gaze: the scientists were part of the goings-on at St Mary's Road.

The fact that the CIAM illustration was reprinted just under 15 years later in the special issue of *Anarchy* mentioned earlier points in the same interpretive direction. It may seem peculiar that an image from the ultimate

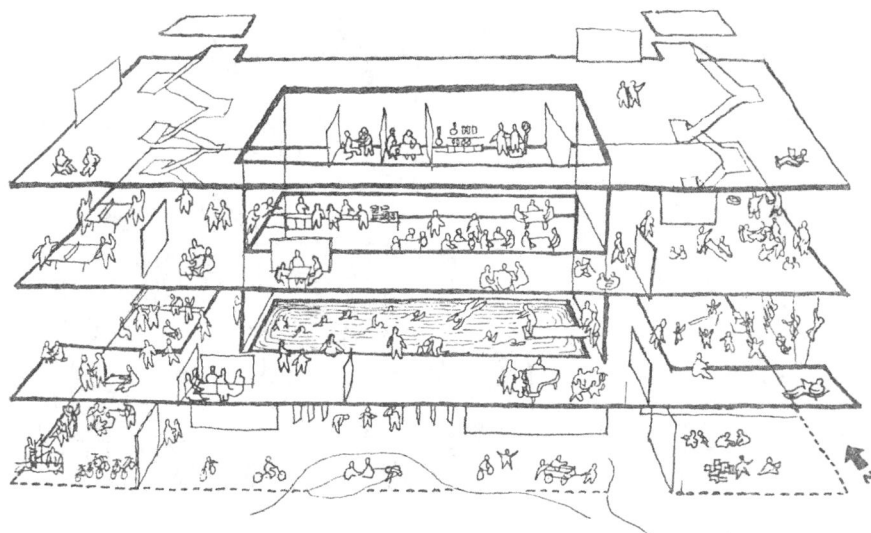

Figure 13.1 Looking through the "bioscope". This drawing is clearly more a product of reading than of personal experience: it engages with a number of narratives and photographs from *The Peckham Experiment*. On its right edge, for example, we see the children playing the famous rope-swinging game on the first floor.
(George Scott Williamson, "The Individual and the Community," in *The Heart of the City: Towards the Humanisation of Urban Life*. CIAM 8/International Congresses for Modern Architecture, ed. Jacqueline Tyrwhitt, José Luis Sert and Ernesto Rogers. Nendeln: Kraus Reprint, 1979 [1952], 30)

planning institution ended up in an anarchists' journal. But it becomes more understandable if we look at the second illustration (Figure 13.2) that the editors of *Anarchy* – including Colin Ward – added to the drawing. In this supplementary illustration the exterior and interior walls have now disappeared entirely, but so have the doctors, biologists, planners, reformers and observers. What is left is a cluster of spontaneously emerging small groups, playfully pursuing various leisure activities.

The experts' gradual disappearance from visual representations of the centre casts light on a broader interpretive context. From the early 1960s on, the Peckham Experiment was increasingly praised by authors who favoured an early form of "advocacy planning".[21] I will mention just one example here. British-American architect and mathematician Christopher Alexander had begun to shift away from the scientism of the older generation of architects and explore approaches that sought to give as many of those affected as possible a say on urban planning decisions. In the wake of this shift he sharply criticized the prescriptive character of neighbourhood planning, though he shared its goal of social integration. In his 1964 book *Notes on the Synthesis of Form*, Alexander, who was inspired by the new

Interpretation

One of the main points they had to consider was flexibility. Movement must not be impeded, because movement is an essential part of the dance of life, and to restrain it is to restrain life. Free circulation and visibility, and the flow of space into space are all necessary qualities of the building. Glass screens set the eye wandering from floor to floor, from activity to activity. The whole building is circulation space and corridors are eliminated. Flexibility could also be achieved by the design of furniture which could be easily moved and handled by those who were to use the building.

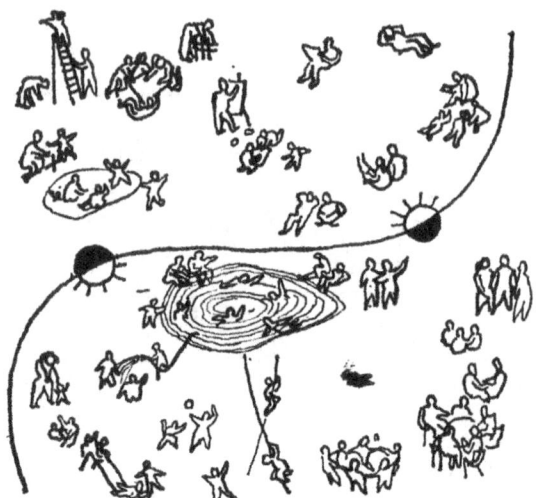

Figure 13.2 The Peckham principle according to *Anarchy*. The "interpretation" alongside the illustration still mentions the building, the free circulation within it and its inspirational glass walls, but we see none of this in the sketch itself. No one appears to be standing back and taking in what is happening; everyone is involved.
(Colin Ward, "Peckham Recollected", *Anarchy* 6 (1966): 55, image detail)

possibilities opened up by computer-aided data-processing, sought to identify so-called "patterns of interaction" in the design process.[22] These he then visualized as diagrams. As Alexander saw it, planning must become reflexive, in other words it must learn to cope with social changes, including those it itself had set in motion. Just under ten years later, Alexander then mentioned the centre in Peckham in his handbook *A Pattern Language*, a publication that points to further shifts in the discourse of planning. Its countercultural emphasis on empowerment is hard to miss: the book is a collection of pieces of advice and little sketches, which are intended to aid the individual design of various buildings. The PHC appears in a section on the topic of the "health center". Here Alexander's advice is that such centres should be geared towards health rather than illness. Above all, though, they must help people become active. In this way health centres might become key nodes within the web of social encounters: sites of the crystallization of small, autonomous communities.[23] It is important to note that Alexander's book summed up the experiences he had accrued in the "Oregon experiment": in 1975 he had been commissioned by the University of Oregon to contribute to the collaborative design of its campus as a so-called "architect-facilitator", as he put it, its brutalist planning having previously led to clashes between students and the university's leadership.[24]

Brave new worlds

The eclectic references anarchists and architects made to the centre may appear to be of marginal significance. But when studied closely they provide evidence of a remarkable shift in the hopes, knowledge and even self-image of elites concerned with social reform in the second half of the twentieth century, particularly in the Anglophone world. This evidence begins to firm up if we consider three visions of the future that referred to the Peckham Experiment at intervals of about ten years.

The year 1947 saw the publication of *Vision in Motion*, the final, post-humously published book by László Moholy-Nagy (who died the year before), a former Bauhaus teacher and former colleague of Gropius who had emigrated to the United States. This influential work – Alexander referred to it in his *Notes* – was a core element in the curriculum of the Institute of Design in Chicago, probably the leading American design school of the post-war era. Moholy-Nagy was convinced that the time was ripe to stimulate the creativity inherent in every human being. A key instrument here was an activating educational approach that would expose people to novel spatio-temporal, indeed kinetic experiences. This could be augmented by an artistic practice combining a variety of media: "[V]ision in motion – is simultaneous grasp. Simultaneous grasp is creative performance – seeing, feeling and thinking in relationships and not as a series of isolated phenomena."[25] Moholy-Nagy backed up his recommendations with a diagnosis of the contemporary world little different from that of Pearse and Scott Williamson. He believed it imperative to counteract the "dangerous antibiological and antisocial dynamics" of a technology-saturated world. Moholy-Nagy too was convinced that the modern "age of isolation" suffered from excessive specialization on the one hand and a widespread alienation from one's work on the other. This, he contended, begins with school education, which fails to arouse a sense of responsibility in pupils. Rather than being "led", however, schoolchildren must engage with the world by "experimenting" – again, the choice of terminology is no coincidence – while simultaneously unleashing their own creative potential.[26] This is where the Peckham Experiment comes into play. Moholy-Nagy presented it as the model of a meeting place capable of stimulating "activity in relationships" and thus engendering "activized social living in the most varied and productive forms of culture and health" – using words that might have been copied directly from the work of Pearse and Scott Williamson. What Moholy-Nagy had in mind here was an inter-disciplinary elite of artists and scientists, who would initially test out such stimuli in a "laboratory" modelled on the centre:

> [I]t could serve as the intellectual trustee of a new age in finding a new unity of purpose; not a life of metaphysical haze but one based upon the biological justice to develop all creative capacities for individual and social fulfilment. It could write a new charter of human life, culminating

in the right for individual and the capacity of self expression (the best bond for social coherence) without censorship or economic pressure. It could translate Utopia into action.[27]

Moholy-Nagy was implacably elitist, however much he may have underlined the need for participation. More importantly, however, his book concluded with the same utopian puzzle that haunts the Peckham writings: what is it that makes the "capacity for fulfilment" the "best bond for social coherence"? Yet, unlike Scott Williamson and Pearse (in whose texts, in case of doubt, the cosmos provided the ultimate justification), Moholy-Nagy highlighted recent research in organizational sociology and social psychology. The aim of good design, he wrote, is the integration of a broad array of factors – of a social, material and technological nature. Hence, by definition designers practise "thinking in relationships", as we read at the start of the book. At the Institute of Design in Chicago, Moholy-Nagy tells us, the capacity for such thinking is already being nurtured in its introductory courses, with the students establishing small, autonomous working groups. The model for these are the novel personality checks being used in the business world. In the social context, he explains, these must be viewed as a means of "self-testing" that teases out individuals' cooperative skills. Finally, Moholy-Nagy asserts that the Institute of Design, in collaboration with the Welfare Department of the state of Illinois, has developed a programme of aptitude tests that reflects the current practice of group therapy[28] – a field of research that we will be taking a closer look at in a moment.

"Peckham" soon lent scientific credibility to other quasi-utopian publications as well, as evident in the work of Aldous Huxley, prominent brother of one of the PHC's leading supporters. In 1958, 11 years after the publication of Moholy-Nagy's book, Huxley assessed the predictive value of his dystopia *Brave New World*, published more than a quarter of a century earlier. In *Brave New World Revisited* Huxley again excoriated dictatorship and mass society and warned of the "nightmare of total organization". He was, however, very much in favour of "positive" social conditioning. While indoctrination is ineffective, Huxley tells us, it is quite possible to influence an individual's social milieu. Every attempt to enforce a rigid behavioural norm, he explains, spawns monsters. Conversely, freedom – which Huxley justifies as a value with reference to human biological diversity – is possible only within a "self-regulating community of freely co-operating individuals". The imperative, then, must be to "break up modern society's merely functional collectives into self-governing, voluntary co-operating groups, capable of functioning outside the bureaucratic systems of Big Business and Big Government". This, we are told, is no fantasy: "[I]n London, the Peckham experiment has demonstrated that it is possible, by co-ordinating health services with the wider interests of the group, to create a true community even in a metropolis."[29]

Finally, more entertaining than Huxley's rather haphazard vision of the future is a 1969 bestseller whose status as science fiction is plain for all to see.

At the heart of the novel *Macroscope* by American Piers Anthony is an instrument of the same name, which, in the near future – the 1980s – is tested out on a spaceship in orbit round the Earth, a collaborative project under the auspices of the United Nations.[30] The macroscope analyses a newly discovered type of wave. In principle this device makes it possible to examine any part of the universe, from a single cell to an entire galaxy. But it also receives transmissions from extra-terrestrial civilizations that perished millions of years ago, including a hypnotic alien interference signal, a fascinating mathematical puzzle that gradually kills the scientists on the spaceship – though it only puts the highly intelligent under its deadly spell. As the plot develops a group of individuals brought together by chance takes possession of the macroscope, heading into deep space as they flee from the UN lackeys who wish to use the device for surveillance. One of the well-intentioned thieves is Anthony's protagonist, Ivo Archer, the product of an educational experiment on earth 20 years earlier. Inspired by the successes of the Peckham Experiment, scientists had allowed selected children to grow up in centres replete with intellectual and musical stimuli. The project had failed; contrary to expectation it had produced just a few geniuses. Archer himself is of only average intelligence, so it appears, which is why use of the macroscope is unable to harm him. However, it is soon revealed that his identity is only the temporary manifestation of the malevolent "Schön", the most intelligent result of the experiment. Schön is just waiting for his shot at world domination. Over time, however, his "host" Archer has developed his own friendly and cooperative personality. It is this that enables Archer and his companions to learn to pool their knowledge and their (emotional, technical and artistic) talents as they flee. After an odyssey through space Archer, equipped with this armoury of social skills, is able to keep Schön under control. The simultaneous unleashing of his full human potential neutralizes the interfering transmitter's effect on him. Humanity now has at its disposal the knowledge of a virtually infinite number of galactic civilizations. Anthony thus uses the centre to ground his narrative historically, rendering it more realistic. But many of the novel's themes also recall the ideas of Pearse and Scott Williamson. The macroscopic perspective, the capacity to see everything at once, including oneself, is akin to the "Peckham" bioscope. Also notable are a certain anti-institutionalism and a rejection of mathematical, isolating thought. Most striking of all, though, is the motif of the complementarity of talents within a heterogeneous constellation of individuals.

But enough of allusions. Moholy-Nagy, Huxley and Anthony, as well as many influential mid-century anarchists and architects, sought to ground their visions of the future in (past) reality by making reference to the centre in Peckham. From a history-of-knowledge standpoint, the basic tenor is the same in all these cases. These authors' expectations were anchored in the internal dynamics of small social groups, dynamics that promised to unlock individuals' latent abilities. For Huxley and Moholy-Nagy in particular the imperative was to trigger these group dynamics, with experts helping to enrich the average person's immediate environment. Their proposals indicate their anxiety over what they saw as the drive-ridden masses' negligible capacity for learning and participation. But they are also a sign of their fears that a state apparatus might manipulate and control the masses. These concerns were no doubt engendered by burgeoning theories of totalitarianism, the "authoritarian personality" and similar tropes that seemed even more pertinent as the Cold War began to take off.

By way of contrast, the ideas developed about the PHC by Christopher Alexander, Colin Ward and Piers Anthony from the mid 1960s on were less pessimistic in character. They too placed their hopes in social groups. In their thinking, however, the specialist played a role, at most, as "facilitator", a role in the literal sense: as a *participant* in a social event. Here "Peckham", as an object of reference, also appreciably changed. The centre finally became the locus of spontaneous self-organization it is known as today. This shift in its interpretation, however, cannot be fully understood without considering the hopes increasingly invested in *psychological* experimentation with human groups in the second half of the twentieth century, to which I will now turn.

A "strange laboratory"?

Polemically put, after 1946 the Pioneer Health Centre was no longer the scene of an experiment but rather of a collective enactment of an experiment. But even the research pursued at the centre during the pre-war period can at most be described as quasi-experimental, if we judge it by the standards of the physiological laboratory experiments carried out by Pearse and Scott Williamson themselves in the early 1930s. Such experiments sought to verify a hypothesis by exercising a systematic influence on predetermined parameters of a natural process. This presupposed a fleshed-out theory; successful experiments had to demonstrate a precise control of variables, must take the form of a series and include the mathematical formalization of their findings. At no time did the Peckham Experiment meet even one of these criteria. Nor was this the directors' aim. Neither of them saw their research project as revealing discrete biological mechanisms in the manner of the scalpel or the addition of chemical reagents. Quite the reverse: it was distinguished by the fact that it established a preserve of "life as a whole".

This might easily prompt us to dismiss the directors' research as pseudoscience. When it comes to the study of knowledge production, however, such ahistorical and normative categories rarely get us anywhere. The anthropology of the laboratory pursued over the last few decades from a history-of-science perspective has shown that even the experimental systems of, say, biochemistry represent highly complex cultural-material hybrids. Certainly, these systems can largely exclude random chance, but it would be quite wrong to think of them as a linear accumulation of evidence. In fact they produce differences, traces or "inscriptions" that are constantly being fed back into the laboratory, modifying the scientists' questions.[31] Most experiments in the natural sciences revolve around hazy "boundary objects"; numerous factors influence the production of these "cognitive artefacts".[32] Among these factors are economic forces, but also material, technological and media-related phenomena: imaging methods, for example, which feature their own ineluctable logics. Finally, guiding concepts, metaphors and narratives play into this process, with scientists retrospectively detaching them from the natural world they have come to understand with their help.

What we find, then, is a blurring of the boundary between experiments in the strict sense and undertakings that may be described as experiments only in a figurative sense. Ultimately the term may mean a pilot project, test, simulation, scenario or even just a project. This perspective opens up a broad comparative field of experimental acts, often of a utopian character. During the time of the Peckham centre, this included insular model communities such as the New Deal housing projects in the United States, with their experiments in cooperation, and the garden cities and artists' communities established by British social reformers.[33] The latter especially were elite self-experiments. They were intended to simultaneously put to the test and showcase a better future society. Often, this was initially explored in fictional form – a famous example being the ideal behaviourist society conceived by B.F. Skinner in his novel *Walden Two* (1948). Hence, we might place "Peckham" somewhere in the middle of a scale with natural scientific experiments at one end and mere thought experiments, even works of fiction, at the other.

These classifications, however, do little to advance our understanding of the promise the Peckham Experiment held for many commentators who were not involved in it. It is more helpful to ask why the term "experiment" suggested itself to the PHC researchers when they presented what they themselves conceded was a rather "strange laboratory"[34] to a broad public – and why so many commentators embraced the notion of Peckham as an experiment as well. The twentieth century was of course generally characterized by a widespread symbolism of experimentation and laboratories – a fact that is undoubtedly due to science's tremendous societal legitimacy but also to the secular experience of social contingency in the modern era.[35] But this observation makes it all the more significant that it was only from the second half of the 1930s onwards that Pearse, Crocker and Scott Williamson began to refer to the Pioneer Health Centre as an experiment. In other words they did so at the very moment they realized how dependent they were on their guinea pigs' involvement. They adopted this terminology as it became apparent that the "biological" processes unfolding at their centre could only be studied through some sort of participant observation. Strikingly, the researchers were thus attracted to the term "experiment" when they publicized findings that were not quantifiable and whose conditions of production were not repeatable. It is hard to assess the risks involved in this choice of term. Hence, if we want to better determine the representativity of the Peckham Experiment, it makes sense to conclude by asking which other research projects, also described as experiments, commentators linked with the centre at the time. To pre-empt the following discussion: not one of these projects was medical in the strict sense of the term.

Northfield, Hawkspur and Hawthorne

A last look at one of Colin Ward's publications provides us with our first piece of evidence. In 1966 the British anarchist published an article examining whether anarchism might be understood as a "theory of social organization". He concluded that it could, citing the Peckham Experiment as scientific proof but also referring to the "theory of the leaderless group".[36] Again, he was pointing to the past in arguing for a better future: the research approach Ward alluded to here had been forged around 25 years earlier, during the Second World War, as a consequence of efforts by the British armed forces to enhance the composition of combat units, partly in order to bolster soldiers' mental resilience. Such units were no longer to be created solely by eliminating the unsuitable but also through prudent allocation of those "personalities" capable of obtaining the best performance from their comrades. This also seemed vital in light of the spread of a new infantry tactic. The hierarchically organized trenches of the last war, which turned soldiers into human materiel, were increasingly superseded by combat between autonomous assault units. Their members' resistance to fatigue and "morale" were both heavily dependent on the affective ties between them and their emotional attachment to the group itself. It was quickly discovered that not every officer was equally good at generating such feelings. The army thus began to rethink the traditional practice of recruiting officers chiefly from the upper classes. Democratization and scientification appeared to dovetail. Against this background the Royal Army Medical Corps and, to an even greater degree, the War Office Selection Board were interested even in unconventional ideas if they promised to make the army fight more effectively. This paved the way for a number of young psychiatrists, often with roots in a European scene dominated by the disciples and admirers of Freud, to think along the lines of what today would be called organizational sociology.

One member of this circle was psychologist Wilfred Bion, inventor of the "leaderless group test", to which Colin Ward alluded. This test was intended to facilitate comparison of officer candidates' leadership qualities, with a form of military role play creating a situation in which their individual desire (to become an officer) compelled them to prove their capacity for cooperation.[37] Not long afterwards Bion began to study group dynamics with a view to their therapeutic potential, and it is here that we can most clearly see parallels with the Peckham Experiment: in the spirit of the recently developed occupational therapy, Bion proposed using everyday social life at the hospital to help heal war trauma. In 1943, together with John Rickman – a former colleague at the Tavistock Clinic in London – he initiated the first of the two so-called Northfield experiments.[38] In a military hospital near Birmingham several hundred soldiers, who were considered psychologically unfit for service, were taken to a wing designated for training. There they were largely left to themselves. The members of this therapeutic community, as it was soon being called, were merely asked to form groups autonomously. They were to organize activities that reflected their interests – woodwork, cartography clubs and the like. Conflicts quickly broke out among the soldiers, highlighting their psychosocial adaptive problems. These problems – this was the only non-negotiable rule – were discussed at the daily roll call, which took on the character of a large-scale therapy session. What Bion and Rickman then observed has a familiar ring to it. Thanks to the soldiers' mutual stimulation the initially passive-chaotic conditions gradually transitioned into a social order. Apparently some of the soldiers even created a cleaning crew off their own bat. The first experiment lasted for just six weeks, the resulting mayhem having sparked protests from the other hospital staff. This, however, did not stop the two psychologists from publishing a much-quoted article shortly afterwards. The topic was so-called "intra-group tensions", but also the therapeutic value of the participants' analysis of these tensions. The article appeared in *The Lancet*, which had also carried many reports on the Peckham Experiment.[39]

Apparently, Rickman, a deft networker and co-founder of the British Psychoanalytical Society who was soon to become a figure of some influence, was not familiar with the centre in Peckham at the time of the first Northfield experiment.[40] By 1944 at the latest, however, he had discussed their observations with Pearse and Scott Williamson in person.[41] We came across Rickman's name earlier: he was a member of the group of scientific advisers consulted by the Health Trust in 1949 in an attempt to help the beleaguered centre. In this role he produced a memorandum on the centre that made a direct connection between it and the findings of the Northfield experiment. The latter, he wrote, made him appreciate the "anthropological" work being done in London.[42] While other experts had objected to the Peckham researchers' lack of objectivity when dealing with users, Rickman saw this as one of the experiment's virtues. In his experience, the memorandum stated, professional scientists were often incapable of adapting to the special conditions of experiments involving people. Among the psychologists in Birmingham, it went on, it was above all the more passionate soldiers who had made their mark. They alone managed to bring their "whole personality" into the community under investigation, and this had made them more acceptable to the soldiers. The centre in Peckham too, he contended, was blessed with investigators "who can deal with people as persons and not only as guinea pigs".

Just under a year after the end of the first experiment Rickman's colleague Harold Bridger, together with psychiatrist S.H. Foulkes, carried out a second experiment in Northfield. By now Pearse and Scott Williamson's theories had become an important reference point in their circle. In the early 1990s Bridger recalled reading *The Peckham Experiment* with great enthusiasm in the run-up to the second experiment; for him, its authors were describing an unwitting experiment in social psychology. It is in fact impossible to miss the parallels between the second Northfield experiment and its Peckham counterpart. Once again the soldiers were encouraged to establish clubs; this time they even published a patients' magazine. In retrospect Bridger described the project as an attempt to create a "hospital-as-a-whole". Influenced by the PHC, he stated, he had a large room declared the Hospital Club and allowed the men themselves to negotiate how it was used. Looking back, rather than a sickbay Bridger regarded the hospital wing as a "space for potential development": "The extensive range of options [...] gives each man every opportunity to satisfy his needs or to test out fantasies. [...] Now he can experiment and test himself out." This gave rise to a "growing [collective] sense of achievement and responsibility".[43] To a greater degree than Bion and Rickman, Bridger and Foulkes believed they had done more than just re-establish a military unit that was fit for action. They had, they thought, also discovered a method for preparing soldiers for peacetime society – in so-called Civil Resettlement Units. But most importantly, Bridger underlined that the psychologists involved had also improved their own social skills. He explained that they – officers, let it be remembered, with the right of command – had learned to stop seeing themselves as sources of authority and instead to think of themselves as part of a community. Here Bridger quoted his colleague Tom Main, who had written in 1946 that it had been far from easy but highly instructive for medics "to renounce [their] power and shoulder social responsibilities".[44] Much like Scott Williamson, then, Bridger believed that the most the psychologists needed to do was to assist in the development of an open-ended dynamic.

It should be noted that the Northfield experimenters also drew on a second source of inspiration, which they retrospectively connected with the centre in London: the so-called Hawkspur experiment of 1936–1940. This project involved a hut camp that delinquent youths had to run by themselves.[45] In the opinion of the camp's main initiator, David Wills, as a result of the great freedoms enjoyed there but also the imperative of cooperation, the adolescents – volunteers and all of them male repeat offenders – had been deprived of the possibility of projecting their self-destructiveness onto authority figures. This had compelled them to explore their own personalities and desires. This in turn, Wills contended, had greatly reduced the rate of recidivism compared with the "borstals" so central to the youth penal system. Wills published this thesis in 1941 in his book *The Hawkspur Experiment*. It is not just the title that recalls the most important book on the Peckham Experiment, which appeared not long afterwards: according to Wills the foregoing of intervention had engendered a constructive "atmosphere of anarchy". He wrote: "[T]he only remedy is to increase the amount of freedom for a spell so that, by learning to control themselves in this greater freedom, the relatively less free atmosphere of normal society will present fewer problems to them."[46]

Providing a third and final clue regarding the place of "Peckham" within the mid-twentieth-century culture of social experimentation, a far better-known series of experiments was also linked with the centre. Like the researchers in London, according to American community physician Kerr Lachlan-White in 1947, the so-called Hawthorne experiments underlined the need to pay greater attention to the "total person in the total situation".[47] I will refrain from going into great detail about these experiments, which have been thoroughly studied by historians of sociology.[48] What matters is that in the 1924–1932 period – around the same time as Scott Williamson and Pearse got together with their experimental participants for the first time on Queen's Road – a series of studies was carried out in the Hawthorne works in Chicago, run by Western Electric, a subsidiary of AT&T. These sought to identify ways of increasing factory workers' productivity. The Chicago researchers initially intended to evaluate methods in the physiology of work and industrial psychiatry (among other things they explored the lighting of work stations). Over the course of their investigations, however, they concluded that these were far less significant to maximizing productivity than the degree of social integration in the workplace. What is striking with regard to the semantics of experimentation in the mid 1930s is that this identification of the so-called "human factor" in the factory was presented as a *chance discovery*. This interpretation was chiefly disseminated by Elton Mayo, founder of the later human relations movement, which was kicked off by the Hawthorne studies.[49] According to Mayo, the Hawthorne scientists had put their faith in a friendly, non-invasive approach to the workers under observation in an attempt to ensure their cooperation in the research. Regardless of the specific productivity-enhancing technique the researchers explored, a small group of women workers (engaged in the assembly of relays), who had undergone various tests, had then become steadily more efficient in their piecework. This, as interviews later revealed, was due to their greater social satisfaction at work. Apparently, a group identity had come into being precisely because the workers had been left to themselves and, above all, because they had seen themselves as part of an experiment. This finding played a major role in the emergence of organizational theory. Henceforth production engineers had to facilitate spontaneous communication within work teams; as a matter of principle these should be put together in such a way as to engender a harmonious internal affective structure. The belief was that this would increase productivity while inspiring far less resistance than the classical Taylorist planning and control of discrete work steps.

Experiments in self-organization

These three examples show that the Peckham Experiment should be seen against the background of a research trend that we might call the experimentalization of social self-organization. The scientific goals and disciplines of the experimenters in London, Birmingham and Chicago differed, of course. And yet, even in the view of contemporaries, their projects had much in common. First, they brought to light potential inherent in the self-administration of so-called small or primary groups: political, pedagogical, military, therapeutic-medical, but also economic potential. Second, the knowledge generated by these projects became manifest in specific situations. It emerged in distinct spaces, which made it easy to compare them with laboratories in the narrow sense of the term: the wing of a hospital, a youth camp and the "test rooms" of the Hawthorne works created exceptional conditions in which rules were suspended. Third, the effects of the interactions between people then observed often exceeded initial expectations. If we are to believe the researchers' reports, these effects even made themselves felt in their own personalities, to their surprise. Fourth, it is striking that this suspension of rules related chiefly to societal spheres traditionally typified by highly vertical structures. From their initiators' perspective, these undertakings became experiments in part because they tentatively abolished hierarchies between doctors and patients, officers and recruits, educators and delinquents, foremen and workers. Ultimately, those involved learned to identify and use resources whose presence was only revealed when traditional institutional and professional barriers had been dismantled.

There is good reason to view this learning effect in light of a broader process of democratization. Empirical studies of social self-organization were undertaken chiefly in the parliamentary democracies of the "West" and they proliferated during the Second World War. Particularly in the UK, experiments in self-organization thus came to the fore at a time when society itself seemed to have become more permeable: through the class-transcending "people's war". Political decision-makers came under pressure to mobilize citizens, but also to tap people's mental energy in order to fight the war more effectively and bolster the war economy. This was accomplished by greatly extending state control of production. But people were also promised increased participation in the future post-war society, the new technique of opinion polling having shown that mere propaganda did little to bolster endurance.[50] The state thus began to highlight the prospect of welfare entitlements and increased democratic participation, in other words political citizenship.[51]

But the growing interest in the functioning of small groups was also bound up with the internal dynamics of the scientification of the social in the 1930s and 1940s. This applies in particular to the "sociologization" of the psy-sciences (and vice versa). Crucially, much of the research in the human sciences during these decades was informed by certain normative assumptions: in view of the perceived potential for conflict in highly stratified societies under simultaneous threat from massification, social experts regarded it as their duty to revive the binding forces diminished by modernization. But even before the war, in an attempt to better understand the mechanisms of adaptation and integration and thus expedite the planning of communities, some social scientists and psychologists had begun to induce social dynamics under the "secure" conditions of the laboratory. In these behavioural experiments the "object and subject of experimentation were identical",[52] because, ultimately, the entities under observation were beings that created meaning; they reflected on their status as guinea pigs. Hence, particularly in those experimental set-ups in which participants could enter into communicative relationships with the experimenters, the latter ran the risk of "channelling the experimental subjects' behaviour in the direction of their hypotheses".[53] In some instances the specialists became aware of these problems and this then impacted deeply on their understandings of society itself.

Mid-century interactional experiments thus contributed to a process in which certain normative assumptions guiding the interpretation of society lost their self-evidence. Essentialist concepts of societal order were superseded by more fluid categories. With increasing frequency society was conceptualized as the ephemeral sum of communicative acts, as the totality of those social "relations" so frequently mentioned in the reception of the PHC. An example that references the Peckham Experiment might help bring this out. The British experiments in military psychology had an American parallel in the sociometry founded by Jacob L. Moreno; from the late 1930s on the sociometrists worked to achieve the mathematical formalization of small groups' internal emotional structures, an approach that led to the development of so-called "buddy ratings" as well as veritable cartograms mapping links between individuals. The American sociometrists too took note of the PHC and they interpreted it in a striking way. In 1945 Maria Rogers reviewed *The Peckham Experiment* in depth for *Sociometry*, the Moreno school's leading organ of publication. In her opinion the London researchers had provided experimental evidence that an environment kept as open as possible could engender "constantly mounting creativity among the members", a "heightened zest for life, readier assumption of responsibilities, more independence of thought and improvement in physical health as well". For Rogers the book had just one flaw: the authors' belief that the processes of improvement they observed could first and foremost be put down to genetic ties. Rogers did not doubt the significance of the biological "family unit" to interpersonal stimulation, as described by Pearse and Crocker. But she explained this significance solely in light of the "formal functions our society has assigned to" this unit. She concluded: "It is, therefore, *relationships* about which the authors are talking throughout the book, and its usefulness would have been greater had this fact been made more explicit."[54] This example puts a crucial thread running through the history of the centre's reception in a nutshell: ironically, their readers could easily disregard the very aspect of their experiment that the Peckham researchers were most interested in – the laws of nature governing human growth. Only the bare bones of the organic "whole" foregrounded in Peckham remained.

Significantly, in much the same way as Pearse and Crocker's "democratized science", experimenting with human relationships also entailed a positive potential of its own, at least for some researchers, namely as a form of social practice. This is particularly evident in the discovery of the so-called "Hawthorne effect", that is, the aforementioned stimulating impact of the experimental situation itself. The very element that might have been viewed as an error within the human scientists' laboratory – lack of distance from the object of investigation – appeared to reveal the enormous potential for inducing social micro-situations.[55] These situations in turn seemed to enable (and press) people to confront their own desires. Ultimately, the self-awareness intensified in this contextual fashion promised to enhance the experimental subjects' sense of responsibility.

This idea too, then, is part of the conceptual history of experimentation in the twentieth century: psychological research on personal responsibility, self-determination and self-organization, carried out around the same time as the Peckham Experiment, correlated with a shift in the semantics of experimenting, which now increasingly encompassed exploratory, playful, creative activities.[56] In sum, these developments help elucidate why, in 1943, the term "experiment" suggested itself to Pearse and Scott Williamson as a way of characterizing a research project that was producing anything but objective data.

Therapeutic experiments

The lessons of the group experiments of the 1930s and 1940s have an interesting history of their own, which is worth telling in brief because it helps us understand some present-day commentators' critical view of the Peckham Experiment. In 1946 Bion and his colleagues established the Tavistock Institute of Human Relations in London, an offshoot of the Tavistock Clinic (the issue of its formal status within the NHS, incidentally, caused quite a headache). These British researchers soon came into close contact with the Research Center for Group Dynamics at the Massachusetts Institute of Technology. Founded in 1945 by Kurt Lewin, a Gestalt psychologist who had emigrated from Germany to the United States, the Research Center was engaged in the experimental exploration of small social groups, studying such things as the effect of different leadership styles on group members' performance and attitudes. Beginning in 1947 the two institutions jointly published the journal *Human Relations*. Since the early 1990s a growing number of analyses have been published on the effects of this transatlantic interdisciplinary cooperation on twentieth-century society: authors like Nikolas Rose believe the knowledge produced by these institutions underpins practices that operationalize the "private self" to create economic value. These practices include techniques of personnel testing and approaches anchored in theories of motivation, methods present to this day in the team evaluations carried out by human resources departments.[57] The "leaderless group discussion", in fact, continues to be used in assessment centres. Significantly, the Tavistock Institute itself was transformed into a consultancy firm over the course of the 1950s and 1960s. Among other things it took on commissioned work for industry, developing so-called "organizational change projects".[58]

But as early as the 1940s social experimentation was also looked upon in a more general sense as a means of creating a more open yet harmonious society. Kurt Lewin in particular viewed his "training groups" or "T-groups" as more than just a form of therapy. He considered them an aid to democratization capable of enhancing participants' self-control, adaptability and capacity for learning.[59] The "T-groups" also showed affinities with the Peckham Experiment in the sense that they promised to produce a kind of artificial state of nature, that is, to eliminate factors such as social background and educational attainment. A *tabula rasa* appeared to have been generated if an initial conflict broke out, for example when group members sought to agree on a collective style of discussion. It was this that created the basis for participants to achieve a shared understanding of the particular way their group functioned. A process was thus set in motion that, so it was believed, could be optimized by analysing the transcripts of discussions, particularly if this analysis itself was later discussed in the group. This example shows once again how deeply Pearse and Scott Williamson had withdrawn into their shaky conceptual edifice after the war: in the 1930s they too had attempted to theoretically penetrate the phenomenon of interpersonal "nurture" – as intensified through an unrestrained flow of information. However, in the following decade they failed to realize that other social experiments increasingly seemed to confirm the existence of a comparable process of enrichment: namely the emancipatory effects triggered when the participants in an experimental group session processed the signals flowing between them and subsequently fed them back into the group.[60]

In any case, in light of this self-referentiality group therapy was well-nigh predestined for linkage with the new lead science that emerged in the late 1940s: cybernetics. The metaphorical application of the concept of feedback in talking therapies was of particular significance here. The social group became a control circuit. By means of constantly updated reports on their internal state, the participants' individual "is values" and the group's collective "ought values" were harmonized. Much like Christopher Alexander's architect, therapists thus lost their function as external observers. They were transformed into "facilitators" who helped optimize the transfer of data within the group, in other words to feed sympathies and aversions back into it in as undistorted a manner as possible. Soon, with the introduction of affordable technological means of feedback such as tape recorders, they became entirely superfluous.

In a parallel process the scientism of social psychology faded, pushed aside by the new emphasis on self-awareness. Perhaps unsurprisingly, given this valorization of grass-roots democracy and egalitarianism, in the 1960s and 1970s group dynamics were adapted "from below". Migrating from the training laboratories to the popular psy-discourse, they began to inform the encounter group movement. A "norm of transparency" was inscribed into these groups; the laying bare of affects seemed good for everyone, part of a process of collective "growth through information".[61] From the perspective of such groups' initiators, spontaneous group dynamics could often expedite both individual-therapeutic and utopian-social goals. In fact, through the experimental process these objectives appeared to coincide.

However, the political dream that group dynamics might liberate society as a whole soon faded amid the general hype over self-realization so characteristic of the emerging "therapy culture".[62] Increasingly, explicit emphasis was placed on techniques of *self*-experimentalization. Fritz Perls's Gestalt therapy provides us with our final example here, not least because it reveals how interwar European theories of holism were transformed into far more pragmatic behavioural advice after crossing the Atlantic. Perls, akin to the Peckham researchers, was influenced by Jan Smuts and, like S.H. Foulkes, had been a student of Weimar holist Kurt Goldstein before emigrating from Nazi Germany to the United States. In 1951, in collaboration with later countercultural theorist and gay rights pioneer Paul Goodman, Perls published an early classic of popular psychology: *Gestalt Therapy* included 18 experiments intended to help people increase their awareness, understood chiefly as an intensified experience of the self (including tips on masturbation). The authors saw their book as inviting readers to go on an "expedition" into their own intimate sphere and, ultimately, to comprehend "self as action".[63] In addition they underlined the need to "include the experimenter in the experiment" in traditional therapeutic situations – an approach that Perls put into practice in subsequent years in his courses for the Esalen Institute at Big Sur in California.[64] The Institute itself is often regarded as the birthplace of the 1970s Californian milieu centred on "finding oneself", a milieu that rapidly opened itself to a diffuse spiritualism and philosophical imports from Asia: yoga, meditation and the like. The psycho-techniques developed on the west coast of the United States soon seeped into the New Age religions with their pronounced faith in self-optimization. Ultimately, in heavily watered-down form, these techniques then flowed into the broader psycho-culture. Again, this brings us back to the present. For in recent times this culture has fallen into disrepute; it seems pervaded by a sense of entitlement, consumerism and an escapism that is detrimental to political life.[65]

The experimental animal

In 1944 Scott Williamson composed an essay entitled "Experimental Living". This is one of his many reinterpretations of the fascinating experiences he accrued a few years earlier at his centre, experiences he subsequently made repeated attempts to get to the heart of – though he never quite managed to do so. Scott Williamson began his text with a critique of contemporary society. We sense his struggle to find an apt expression to describe a species that fails to tap its own inherent potential. Scott Williamson first envisages modern man asleep and lost in daydreams before coming up with an appropriate image: artificial anaesthesia. "We do not live, we sleep and dream. [...] Feelings become anesthetised, and living becomes recumbent star-gazing."

The question is: "Must this be so?" For Scott Williamson there could be no doubt: "We can only find an answer by experiment – by experimenting with people and things." So the Pioneer Health Centre had been created, whose laboratory conditions, the reader learns, can be summed up in a few words: "[E]verybody was absolutely free to do as they felt – to act in accordance with their tastes, feelings, likes and loves. There must be literally no rules within the scientists' laboratory."[66]

This is Scott Williamson's usual ex-post experimentalization, one of his many retrospective attempts to explain his intentions – evident in the above quotation in the shift from the imperfect to the modal. The imagery with which he went on to describe the process of nature – which he believed he had observed in this laboratory – was not new either. The participants in the Peckham Experiment began to turn off the autopilot, he wrote; they overcame the deadening effect of artificial external influences (he mentioned aspirin and Hollywood films); after a year they had learned to operate beyond the routes and routines laid down by society: "They were free of the road, the social highway. They were all experimenting with living."[67]

Then, however, the text takes an odd turn. Scott Williamson concedes – in fact presents it as one of its strengths – that his laboratory had eliminated the difference between the researchers and the objects they studied. Not only does he describe his guinea pigs' unimpeded self-exploration with the same term as his own research project (they *experimented* with life), but goes one step further. He adds that while the scientists at the centre experimented with other people, they had been thoroughly infected by these people's activities: "[A]s a matter of fact, he [the scientist] was just as busy experimenting with his own living – living is very, very infectious and contagious."[68] Scott Williamson has the experiment take on a life of its own. It becomes the true cause of dynamics that had not been foreseen when it began. Once again his essay highlights the fact that in the mid 1930s, together with his partner Pearse, he had entered the Pioneer Health Centre as a typical concerned citizen – emerging after a decade completely transformed: as a researcher among researchers.

Of course, we cannot take his claims of a levelling process at face value. But neither should we dismiss the impression they made on his readers. In fact the above-cited passage helps explain why the Peckham Experiment held such fascination for later commentators in another respect as well. The previous chapter reconstructed how the memory of "Peckham" meandered through the second half of the twentieth century, particularly in Britain. I have shown how it changed constantly as it did so and – most importantly – that it was always mentioned at moments when the priority was to ground the possibility of a better world in real history, as it were. This makes it clear why the sudden, unexpected emergence of order at the centre is such a crucial component of the Peckham legend: for a brief moment, as those who rediscovered the centre believed, it had brought the artifice of historical reason out into the light. It had allowed a glimpse of a happier future.

At the Pioneer Health Centre in Peckham Innes Pearse and George Scott Williamson learned to see the harmonious yet adaptable organic community they secretly wished to perceive. As this book has demonstrated, it is easy to locate their motives in the crisis discourse that marked the centre's early days. But while searching for the mechanism that had transformed the mayhem bedevilling the centre into a lively community within just a few months, the Peckham researchers came across something new: human beings' self-determined and exploratory attitude towards life. Ultimately, of course, those behaviours the researchers recognized among users as a state of nature were ones they themselves had displayed – and thus fed back into the centre. This, however, did not keep them from viewing themselves as experimenting not just with other people but also alongside them.

This assessment itself may well have been powerful enough to blur certain social status boundaries in the district of Peckham. But there is nothing humble about it. When planning the centre its future directors had worked on the assumption that they were going to create ideal conditions for cultivating an ethos of personal responsibility in others. Instead – reinforced by their propensity to view everything through the lens of biology – their scientific habitus became anthropologized. This very operation, however, blinded them to the fact that what social scientists today call cultural, symbolic and economic capital was still distributed in highly unequal fashion at the centre. The forces governing its members' lives could not simply be locked out of the laboratory; social asymmetries determining their behaviour did not vanish as soon as the "guinea pigs" entered the building on St Mary's Road. Instead they were overlaid by another, more subtle asymmetry: a knowledge differential. But the pressure this imposed on participants was not channelled towards specific standards of achievement set by outside authorities. What was expected of entirely normal people in Peckham, perhaps for the first time in such an unambiguous way, was more abstract: they were expected to want to know more about themselves.

More than a few of the centre members were capable of absorbing this pressure and using it productively to their own ends; they lived better lives thanks to "Peckham". In historical perspective, it would generally be quite wrong to hold Pearse, Crocker and Scott Williamson, their colleagues or even their later admirers responsible for the narcissistic culture of therapy or the complementary trend towards self-exploitation so typical of the modern workplace. Nonetheless, I believe, the history of the Peckham Experiment – and the experimental culture within the human sciences of its era – can give us a more nuanced understanding of norms of flexibility in past and present. In looking at the centre and its legacy, we can discern an often overlooked ideal that has at least helped pave the way for the emergence of the enterprising subject (Nikolas Rose), the permanent project worker (Luc Boltanski) or trainer (Peter Sloterdijk) of the contemporary self. Here, an *experimental self* was formed that can be defined by its continual exploration of its own potential. But the history of the Pioneer Health Centre in London also shows that this idealized image of the human being has roots that are not well conveyed, and that stretch back further than suggested, by the narrative of the rise of *homo oeconomicus* after the golden age of the welfare state. The experimental self was certainly moulded and naturalized by the economic theory of utility optimization developed in the late twentieth century. But it was also shaped by socio-biological ideas formulated during the interwar period concerning health, natural potential and the societal prerequisites for their realization. In 1943 Pearse and Crocker had already captured this image in passing in an ambiguous formula, when they referred to the human being as an "experimental animal".[69]

Notes

1 Hebert Read, "The Peckham Experiment", *The Listener* (December 23, 1943): 729. Arrangements were made for Read to meet the PHC directors: Read to Pearse, December 5, 1943, WL, SA/PHC/E.3/11–16.
2 Read to Morgan, November 28, 1943, WL, SA/PHC/E.3/11–16.
3 J.R.M. Brumwell to Scott Williamson, March 19, 1945, WL, SA/PHC/D.2/12.
4 Herbert Read, The Sociology of Imponderables, undated [1945], WL, SA/PHC/D.2/12, 3, 9.
5 Untitled manuscript, undated [1945], WL, SA/PHC/D.2/12.
6 John Hewetson, "Peckham Health Experiment", *Freedom* (1947).
7 David Goodway, "Anarchism and the welfare state: the Peckham Health Centre", *History & Policy* (May 1, 2007), www.historyandpolicy.org/papers/policy-paper-55.html (accessed December 17, 2017).
8 Autarchy at Peckham, 1951, WL, SA/PHC/D.2/20.
9 Colin Ward, "'A laboratory of anarchy'. A comparative anthology", *Anarchy* 6 (1966): 52.
10 Colin Ward, "Fringe benefits", *New Statesman & Society* 213, no. 5 (1992): 26.
11 Donaldson, *Child of the Twenties*, 154. The praise was mutual: around the same time Jack and Frances Donaldson commissioned Gropius to design a country house, having sought the advice of Pearse and Scott Williamson when they perused his plans. Gropius also expressed his fascination with their experiment in a letter to influential Swiss art historian Sigfried Giedion. Gropius to Giedion, February 14, 1935, BAB, Nachlass Walter Gropius, 12/505–506.
12 The Museum of Modern Art, *Modern Architecture in England. With essays by Henry-Russell Hitchcock and Catherine K. Bauer* (New York: Museum of Modern Art, 1937).
13 Clive B. Fenton, "PLAN. A student journal of ambition and anxiety", in *Man-Made Future: Planning, Education and Design in Mid-Twentieth-Century Britain*, ed. Ian Boyd Whyte (London/New York: Routledge, 2007), 188–189.
14 "The Basis of Planning", 182, 184, 186. By this point in time the Peckham directors had also contributed indirectly to the dissemination of New Building. In 1933 Mozelle Sassoon (heir to the Ed Sassoon trading company) asked the PHC executive committee whether there was land available in the vicinity of the PHC where housing reformer Elizabeth Denby and architect Maxwell Fry could build housing. The committee did in fact transfer part of the property on St Mary's Road to the Pioneer Housing Trust. The following year saw the construction of small modern flats with rationalized kitchens and variable room sizes on the site: Darling, *Reforming Britain*, 67.
15 Kuchenbuch: *Geordnete Gemeinschaft.*

16 Pearse and Crocker, *The Peckham Experiment*, 70. In a 1940 radio debate influential urban planning theorist Thomas Sharp extolled the PHC as a template for the nuclei of future neighbourhoods: *The Listener* (1940), 816. In the late 1940s, meanwhile, Kenneth Barlow made an attempt to build a housing estate in Coventry with a health centre at its core. He founded the Family Health Club Housing Association, whose members, in collaboration with architects, were to design their own residences – an early example of participatory planning: Kenneth Barlow, *A home of their own* (London: Faber & Faber, 1946). Despite backing from prominent individuals – including Lewis Mumford: "Town Planning that aims at Health and Happiness", *Coventry Evening Telegraph* (July 5, 1946) – the project came to grief due to the costs and lack of interest on the part of the relevant authorities: Stefan Couperus, "Experimental planning after the Blitz. Non-governmental planning initiatives and post-war reconstruction in Coventry and Rotterdam, 1940–1955", *Journal of Modern European History 13*, no. 4 (2015): 516–533.

17 See for example Jacqueline Tyrwhitt, "Introduction", in *Cities in Evolution*, ed. Patrick Geddes (London: Williams and Norgate, 1949), x.

18 "No speech of the Congress was followed more attentively than the address of Dr Scott Williamson": Sigfried Giedion, undated manuscript [1951], gta, Giedion, 42-SG-36.

19 George Scott Williamson, "The Individual and the Community", in *The Heart of the City: Towards the Humanisation of Urban Life. CIAM 8/International Congresses for Modern Architecture*, eds Jacqueline Tyrwhitt, José Luis Sert and Ernesto Rogers (Nendeln: Kraus Reprint, 1979), 33.

20 It was apparently made by architecture students at the AA School: Tyrwhitt to Scott Williamson and Pearse, September 3, 1951, gta, Jaqueline Tyrwhitt, 42-JT-3-130/424.

21 See the references in Leo Kuper, "Blueprint for Living together", in *Living in Towns. Selected Research Papers in Urban Sociology of the Faculty of Commerce and Social Science University of Birmingham*, ed. Leo Kuper (London: Cresset Press, 1953), 179; and Lawrence Haworth, *The Good City* (Bloomington: Indiana University Press, 1963), 126–128.

22 Christopher Alexander, *Notes on the Synthesis of Form* (Cambridge, Mass.: Harvard University Press, 1964), 3.

23 Christopher Alexander et al., *A Pattern Language. Towns. Buildings. Construction* (New York: Oxford University Press, 1977), 252–255.

24 Christopher Alexander, *The Oregon Experiment. An Essay on the Art of Building and the Nature of the Universe* (New York: Oxford University Press, 1975).

25 László Moholy-Nagy, *Vision in Motion* (Chicago: Paul Theobald & Co 1947), 11.

26 Ibid., quotations: 13, 15, 23, 25.

27 Ibid., 359.

28 Ibid., 42, 72.

29 Aldous Huxley, *Brave New World Revisited* (New York: Harper & Brothers, 1958), 4–5, 120, 8, 141, 143.

30 Piers Anthony, *Macroscope* (New York: Avon Books, 1969).

31 For an example that builds on the work of Bruno Latour, see Hans-Jörg Rheinberger and Michael Hagner, "Experimentalsysteme", in *Die Experimentalisierung des Lebens. Experimentalsysteme in den biologischen Wissenschaften 1850/1950*, eds Hans-Jörg Rheinberger and Michael Hagner (Berlin: Akademie Verlag, 1993), 11–12.

32 Tanner, "'Weisheit des Körpers' und soziale Homöostase", 159.

33 Dennis Hardy, *Utopian England. Community Experiments 1900–1945* (London: E & FN Spon, 2000).

34 Pearse and Crocker, *The Peckham Experiment*, 48.

35 This is why historians too are partial to the metaphor of the laboratory as they seek to capture the nature of modern societies. Their aim here is to bring out the fact that – whatever their differences – these societies can be defined in light of the scientification of knowledge about them, and by an intensified collective sense of possibility.

36 Colin Ward, "The organization of anarchy", in *Patterns of Anarchy. A Collection of Writings on the Anarchist Tradition*, eds Leonard I. Krimerman and Lewis Perry (New York: Anchor Books, 1966), 349–351.

37 Amy L. Fraher, *A history of group study and psychodynamic organizations* (London: Free Association Books, 2004), 48–59.

38 On what follows see Tom Harrison, *Bion, Rickman, Foulkes and the Northfield Experiments: Advancing on a Different Front* (London: Jessica Kingsley Publishers, 2000); and the contributions in Malcom Pines, ed., *Bion and Group Therapy* (London: Jessica Kingsley Publishers, 2000).

39 Wilfred R. Bion and John Rickman, "Intra-group tensions in therapy: Their study as the task of the group", *The Lancet* (November 27, 1943): 678–681. The article also impressed a Frenchman who had himself worked in military psychiatry during the war and who was soon to become a highly fashionable theorist: Jacques Lacan, "English Psychiatry and the War", *Psychoanalytical Notebooks of the London Circle* 4 (2000): 15–19.

40 Harrison, *Bion, Rickman, Foulkes and the Northfield Experiments*, 72–73.

41 The three of them having dined together, Pearse wrote Rickman a letter in which she expressed her delight that he understood and appreciated their research: Pearse to Rickman, November 27, 1944, BPS, Rickman Papers, P03/B/B/03-1.

42 Memorandum on a proposed Research Institute of Human Biology, with reference also to the Peckham Health Centre, November 1949, BPS, Rickman Papers, P03/B/B/03-2.

43 Harold Bridger, "The Discovery of the Therapeutic Community. The Northfield Experiments", in *The Social Engagement of Social Science (SESS). A Tavistock Anthology. Vol. 1: The Socio-psychological perspective*, eds Eric Trist and Hugh Murray (Philadelphia: University of Pennsylvania Press, 1990), 68–87, quotes on 76, 78.

44 Ibid., 82.

45 Malcolm Pines, "Large Groups and Culture", in *The large group re-visited: the herd, primal horde, crowds and masses*, eds Stanley Schneider et al. (London: Jessica Kingsley Publishers, 2003), 47; and Harrison, *Bion, Rickman, Foulkes and the Northfield Experiments*, 26–27.

46 David W. Wills, *The Hawkspur Experiment. An Informal Account of the Training of Wayward Adolescents* (London: Allen and Unwin, 1941), 39, 46. As it happens, in his book Wills put forward very little numerical data to substantiate his claims, so he had to rely on anonymous case studies, including passages explicitly flagged up as fictional. Wills, incidentally, made no secret of the fact that he would give the boys a clip around the ear if things got out of hand: 87.

47 Kerr Lachlan White, "Recent Contributions to the Science of Health", *McGill Medical Journal* (October 1947): 378. Colin Ward also saw these parallels: Ward, *The organization of anarchy*. As early as 1944 an article in the *Listener* had put forward similar arguments, reporting on the new interest in social issues in American psychology: "[The] flowering of potentiality comes about through happy social relationships. [...] The subject [...] links up to the work of Mayo and Whitehead in the field of Industrial Psychology, and with the findings of the Peckham Experiment." C.M. Fleming, "The Social Psychology of Education", *The Listener* (May 4, 1944).

48 On what follows, see Emil Walter-Busch, *Das Auge der Firma. Mayos Hawthorne-Experimente und die Harvard Business School, 1900–1960* (Stuttgart: F. Enke, 1989).
49 Elton Mayo, "Foreword", in *Management and the Worker. Technical vs. Social Organization in an Industrial Plant*, eds Fritz Jules Roethlisberger and William J. Dickson (Cambridge, Mass.: Harvard University Press, 1934), iii–vi.
50 Nick Hubble, *Mass Observation and Everyday Life. Culture, History, Theory* (Basingstoke: Palgrave Macmillan, 2006).
51 See David Morgan and Mary Evans, *The battle for Britain. Citizenship and ideology in the Second World War* (London/New York: Routledge, 1993).
52 Birgit Griesecke et al., "Vorwort", in *Kulturgeschichte des Menschenversuchs im 20. Jahrhundert*, eds Birgit Griesecke et al. (Suhrkamp, 2009), 9.
53 Nicolas Pethes, "Einleitung", in: *Menschenversuche. Eine Anthologie 1750–2000*, ed. Nicolas Pethes (Frankfurt: Suhrkamp, 2008), 722.
54 Rogers, "The Peckham Experiment", 95–96.
55 In fact, the Hawthorne effect soon came to refer chiefly to flawed procedures in social experiments. However, even the more strictly managed control group experiments of the 1960s were not immune to reading their own heuristic models into the behaviour of experimental subjects as normative reality: the experimental set-ups of the 1960s designed to illuminate the aforementioned "authoritarian personality" – such as the famous Milgram experiment – have been interpreted as "postmodern" because they were allegorical dramatizations of moral hypotheses: Augustine Brannigan, "The Postmodern Experiment. Science and Ontology in Experimental Social Psychology", *British Journal of Sociology* 48 (1997): 594–610.
56 Griesecke, "Vorwort", 9.
57 Nikolas Rose, *Governing the Soul. The Shaping of the Private Self* (London: Routledge, 1990). For a sceptical take on Rose's generalizations, see Mathew Thomson, *Psychological Subjects. Identity, Culture, and Health in Twentieth Century Britain* (Oxford: Oxford University Press, 2006). On the broader context see also the recent work by Michal Shapira, *The War Inside: Psychoanalysis, Total War, and the Making of the Democratic Self in Postwar Britain* (Cambridge: Cambridge University Press, 2015).
58 One example of its work is the "Glacier Metal" study, a conflict resolution strategy deployed in the company of the same name, which proposed the creation of largely autonomous working groups. This study updated one of the main suggestions put forward in the context of the Hawthorne experiments: that productivity in the business enterprise and individual emotional enrichment are by no means mutually exclusive concepts: Nikolas Rose and Peter Miller, "The Tavistock Programme: The Government of Subjectivity and Social Life", *Sociology* 22 (1988): 171–192.
59 Ulrich Bröckling, "Über Feedback. Anatomie einer kommunikativen Schlüssel-technologie", in *Die Transformation des Humanen. Beiträge zur Kulturgeschichte der Kybernetik*, eds Michael Hagner and Erich Hörl (Frankfurt: Suhrkamp, 2008), 326–347.
60 Conversely, in 1950 Michael Chance, the aforementioned critical ex-colleague, while underlining that this had not been done consistently in Peckham, contended that it makes sense to render people's interpersonal relationships transparent to them, mentioning the example of the Peckham family consultation. This, he claimed, had been demonstrated by American sociologists: Chance, "Where from Peckham?", 727. Perhaps Pearse and Scott Williamson had missed out an intermediate step. In the early 1930s they had already failed to notice the proto-communication theory being developed by their colleagues in the life sciences. Walter Cannon's "wisdom of the body" would surely have been of interest to them: Cannon underlined the organism's capacity to adapt to changes in its environment in order to survive and its ability to stabilize itself through the communicative

interplay of its component parts. Influenced by the discourse of crisis so prevalent during the interwar period, he perceived the flexibility of the democratic political system as structurally analogous to homeostasis in a healthy body. Stephen J. Cross and William R. Albury, "Walter B. Cannon, L. J. Henderson and the Organic Analogy", *Osiris* 2 (1987): 165–192.

61 Bröckling, "Über Feedback", 336–337.

62 The term was coined by Frank Furedi, *Therapy culture: Cultivating vulnerability in an uncertain age* (London: Routledge, 2004), who argues unconvincingly that the answer is a return to stoicism.

63 Frederick S. Perls, Ralph Hefferline and Paul Goodman, *Gestalt Therapy. Excitement and Growth in the Human Personality* (New York: Dell, 1951), 365.

64 Marion S. Goldman, *The American Soul Rush: Esalen and the Rise of Spiritual Privilege* (New York: New York University Press, 2012); and Linda Sargent Wood, *A More Perfect Union. Holistic Worldviews and the Transformation of American Culture after World War II* (New York/Oxford: Oxford University Press, 2010), 169–198. The Institute received support from Aldous Huxley, who was now considered a pioneer of the "human potential movement".

65 For a representative example that is nonetheless worth seeing, see Adam Curtis's BBC Four documentary *Century of the Self* (2002).

66 Experimental Living, 1944, SA/PHC/D.2/6, 1–2.

67 Ibid., 3.

68 Ibid., 7.

69 Pearse and Crocker, *The Peckham Experiment*, 22.

14 Epilogue

Early September 2011, Peckham in the drizzle, half an hour by bus from Victoria Station. Typical South London, a bit run-down; modest, mostly two-storey buildings. Unremarkable Victorian terraced houses alternate with social housing of brick and concrete built between the 1930s and 1970s. Between them lie patches of waste ground around train tracks and railway bridges. Rather at odds with this setting, I find the former Pioneer Health Centre fenced off, the premises turned into flats, a gated community. A friendly resident arrives and lets me into the grounds, though not the building. Still, I can walk around the – now listed – former centre, in front of which there are parking spaces and a small tennis court. The exterior is well preserved. The delicate window frames and the gutters have suffered, but the facade was painted not too long ago. Colour-wise this is a highly modernist ensemble with a somehow hygienic air: white, surrounded by green, the only striking detail on the facade a lurid yellow alarm. The building still seems purely functional; indeed, it looks like a factory. Only at the rear does it make a more intimate impression, with balconies screened by reed panels featuring barbecues, garden furniture and tree ferns in hefty clay pots. Through the windows one can make out bright, loft-like spaces, designer lamps and eclectic ensembles of furniture, an expensive racing bike – no question, the people who live here care about matters of style.

On the site of a progressive interwar reform project a colony very typical of contemporary London appears to have formed, one pervaded by self-fashioning processes. Is it possible to accumulate prestige by living in a modernist icon steeped in history, a future from the past? I will leave it to others to assess the extent to which this reflects my own interest in the Peckham Experiment. A few weeks later, back in Berlin, I am telling a friend of a friend about my trip to the archives and she mentions that someone told her of an acquaintance living in a converted health centre in South London.

Just under a year later – back in England for follow-up research – Simon lets me into the building. Little "aha" moments ensue: the ceilings are lower than I expected. When I look through the pane of glass on the second floor down to the swimming pool, which is still being used, history comes alive. Large drops of condensed water detach themselves from the

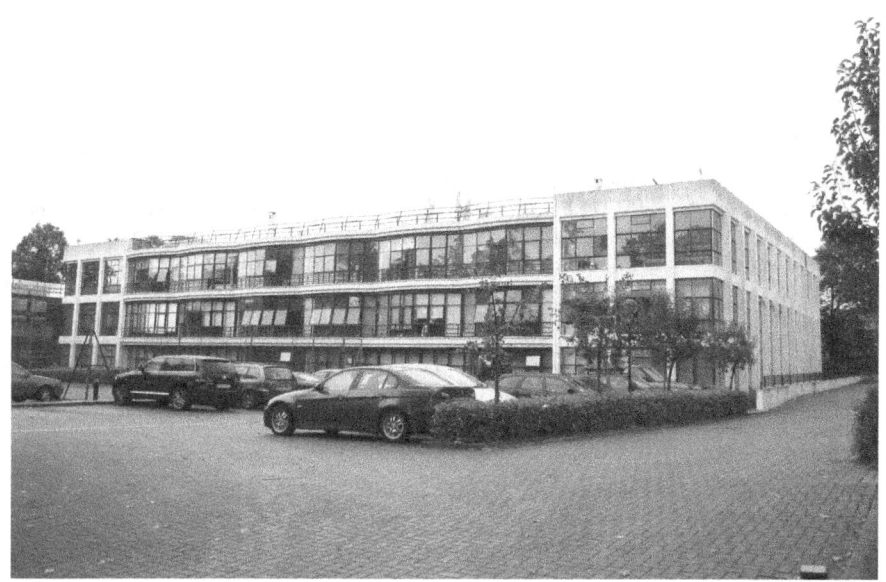

Figure 14.1 St Mary's Road, Peckham, September 4, 2011
(Photograph by the author)

glass roof and fall into the pool, adding to the special atmosphere. It is
not hard to imagine this window framing a snapshot of life for Scott
Williamson and Pearse. The building's conversion into apartments in 2000
was carried out in a respectful way, which explains the air of history. In
fact the company responsible incorporates the building's history into its
marketing. It is now known as the Pioneer Centre; a number of framed
photographs of everyday scenes at the centre in the 1940s adorn the walls
of the ground-floor hallway.[1] Simon himself lives in an apartment on the
top floor with two flatmates (one of whom collects the books of Pearse
and Scott Williamson), evidently where one of the doctors' offices used to
be. Almost all his friends have moved to Peckham from the East End over
the last few years, Simon tells me, partly because the small single-family
houses in the area are popular among young parents. There has, he goes
on, been an appreciable increase in rents and house prices in Peckham.
The residents of the Pioneer Centre itself are mostly members of the
creative class, he states, corroborating my assumption. But it turns out
that things are more complicated than this. Simon is lucky; he and his
flatmates rent the flat cheaply from the owner, who apparently purchased
it for about £350,000, used to live there himself and is unwilling to part
with it for sentimental reasons. In passing I learn of tensions between
owners and renters that have erupted into a war of words on the building's

own Facebook page. It is perhaps fair to say that social inequality is still manifest in "Peckham", though in a very subtle way.

Note

1 There is also a plaque mounted on the fence that commemorates the experiment and an aluminium sculpture near the entrance, which is evidently meant to represent a child in a pram and its parents. The PHC remains quite present in the district's collective memory. For example, near the former centre there was until recently an (apparently very poor) Peckham Experiment Restaurant. The Pioneer Health Foundation mentioned earlier, meanwhile, often organizes events in the area. Two neighbourhood networks have also explored the history of the PHC: "Peckham Residents' Network", http://peckhamresidents.wordpress.com/ and "Peckham Vision", www.facebook.com/PeckhamVision/ (accessed December 17, 2017). The PHC is, of course, mentioned in the district's official chronicle (John D. Beasley, *The Story of Peckham and Nunhead* (London, 1976), esp. 64–68). Even the English-language *Wikipedia* entry on Peckham refers to the centre: "Peckham", http://en.wikipedia.org/wiki/Peckham (accessed December 17, 2017).

References

Aldous, Christopher, and Akihito Suzuki. *Reforming Public Health in Occupied Japan, 1945–52: Alien Prescriptions?* London, New York: Routledge, 2012.

Alexander, Christopher. *Notes on the Synthesis of Form.* Cambridge, Mass.: Harvard University Press, 1964.

Alexander, Christopher. *The Oregon Experiment. An Essay on the Art of Building and the Nature of the Universe.* New York: Oxford University Press, 1975.

Alexander, Christopher, et al. *A Pattern Language. Towns. Buildings. Construction.* New York: Oxford University Press, 1977.

Alexander, Sally. "A New Civilization? London Surveyed 1928–1940s." *History Workshop* 65(2007): 297–320.

Allen, J. "An Experiment in Health." *Health* 5, no. 1(1937): 6–8.

Anker, Peder. *Imperial Ecology. Environmental Order in the British Empire.* Cambridge, MA: Harvard University Press, 2001.

Anthony, Piers. *Macroscope.* New York: Avon Books, 1969.

Armstrong, David. "The Rise of Surveillance Medicine." *Sociology of Health & Illness* 17, no. 3(1995): 393–404.

Ash, Mitchell G. *Gestalt Psychology in German Culture 1890–1967. Holism and the Quest for Objectivity.* Cambridge: Cambridge University Press, 1995.

Baldwin, Peter. *Contagion and the State in Europe.* New York: Cambridge University Press, 2005.

Barlow, Kenneth. *A Home of their Own.* London: Faber & Faber, 1946.

Barlow, Kenneth. "The Peckham Experiment." *Medical History* 29(1985): 264–271.

Barlow, Kenneth. *Recognising Health.* London: McCarrison Society, 1988.

Beach, Abigail. "Forging a 'Nation of Participants'. Political and Economic Planning in Labour's Britain." In *The Right to Belong. Citizenship and National Identity in Britain, 1930–1960*, edited by Abigail Beach and Richard Weight, 98–115. London: I.B. Tauris, 1998.

Beach, Abigail. "Potential For Participation: Health Centres and the Idea of Citizenship c. 1920–1940." In *Regenerating England. Science, Medicine and Culture in Interwar-Britain*, edited by Christopher Lawrence and Anna K. Mayer, 203–230. Amsterdam: Rodopi, 2000.

Beasley, John D. *The Story of Peckham and Nunhead.* London: London Borough of Southwark, 1999.

Bedwell, C.E.A. "With the Hospitals in Britain." *The Canadian Hospital* (May 1946): 50.

Benney, Mark. "The Lost Chord." *International Women's News* (February 1944): 52–53.

Berg, Leila. "Moving towards Self Government." In *Children's Rights. Towards the Liberation of the Child*, edited by Julian Hall, 8–53. London: Panther, 1972a.

Berg, Leila. *Look at Kids*. Harmondsworth: Penguin, 1972b.

Berridge, Virginia. *Health and Society in Britain since 1939*. New York: Cambridge University Press, 1999.

Bion, Wilfred R., and John Rickman. "Intra-group tensions in therapy: Their study as the task of the group." *The Lancet* (November 27, 1943): 678–681.

Blackwell, Gordon W. "The Peckham Experiment." *American Sociological Review* 12 (1947): 259–260.

Blake, Casey Nelson. *Beloved Community. The Cultural Criticism of Randolph Bourne, Van Wyck Brooks, & Lewis Mumford*. Chapel Hill/London: University of North Carolina Press, 1990.

Boltanski, Luc, and Ève Chiapello. *The New Spirit of Capitalism*. London/New York: Verso, 2005 [1999].

Borsay, Anne, and Peter Shapley, eds. *Medicine, Charity and Mutual Aid. The Consumption of Health and Welfare in Britain, c. 1550–1950*. Aldershot: Ashgate, 2007.

Brannigan, Augustine. "The Postmodern Experiment. Science and Ontology in Experimental Social Psychology." *British Journal of Sociology* 48(1997): 594–610.

Brewer, Herbert. "Science, Synthesis and Sanity." *Eugenics Review* 58, no. 1(1966): 33.

Bridger, Harold. "The Discovery of the Therapeutic Community. The Northfield Experiments." In *The Social Engagement of Social Science (SESS). A Tavistock Anthology. Vol. 1: The Socio-psychological Perspective*, edited by Eric Trist and Hugh Murray, 68–87. Philadelphia: University of Pennsylvania Press, 1990.

Bröckling, Ulrich. "Über Feedback. Anatomie einer kommunikativen Schlüsseltechnologie." In *Die Transformation des Humanen. Beiträge zur Kulturgeschichte der Kybernetik*, edited by Michael Hagner and Erich Hörl, 326–347. Frankfurt: Suhrkamp, 2008.

Bröckling, Ulrich, Susanne Krasmann and Thomas Lemke. "From Foucault's Lectures at the Collège de France to Studies of Governmentality. An Introduction." In *Governmentality. Current Issues and Future Challenges*, edited by Ulrich Bröckling, Susanne Krasmann and Thomas Lemke, 1–33. London: Routledge, 2011.

Chance, Michael. "The Peckham Experiment: An Assessment." *Woman Health Officer* (August 1948).

Chance, Michael. "Where from Peckham?" *The Lancet* (April 15, 1950): 726–727.

Charkin, Emily. *"He swings where there is space": Education, Freedom and Community at the Peckham Health Centre 1945–1950*. MA thesis, Institute of Education, University of London, 2010.

Cherry, Steven. "Medicine and Public Health, 1900–1939." In *A Companion to Early Twentieth Century Britain*, edited by Christopher John Wrigley, 405–423. Blackwell: Oxford, 2003.

Child, John. "Quaker Employers and Industrial Relations." *Sociological Review* 12 (1964): 293–315.

Collini, Stefan. *Public Moralists. Political Thought and Intellectual Life in Britain 1850–1930*. Oxford: Oxford University Press, 1991.

Comerford, John. *Health the Unknown. The Story of the Peckham Experiment*. London: Hamish Hamilton, 1947.

Comfort, Alex. "Comes the Revolution." *New Scientist* (December 2, 1965).

Conford, Philip. *The Origins of the Organic Movement*. Edinburgh: Floris Books, 2001.

Conford, Philip. "'Smashed by the National Health?'. A Closer Look at the Demise of the Pioneer Health Centre, Peckham." *Medical History* 60, no. 2(2016): 250–269.

Cottam, David. "Pioneer Health Centre." In *Sir Owen Williams 1890–1969*, edited by David Cottam, 95–100. London: Architectural Association Publications, 1986.

Couperus, Stefan. "Experimental Planning after the Blitz. Non-governmental Planning Initiatives and Post-war Reconstruction in Coventry and Rotterdam, 1940–1955." *Journal of Modern European History* 13, no. 4(2015): 516–533.

Cross, Stephen J., and William R. Albury. "Walter B. Cannon, L. J. Henderson and the Organic Analogy." *Osiris* 2(1987): 165–192.

Cunningham, Hugh. *The Children of the Poor. Representations of Childhood since the Seventeenth Century*. Oxford/Cambridge, MA: Blackwell, 1991.

Danneskiold-Samsøe, Otto. "Peckham-experimentet." *Byggmästaren* 28(1949): 321–326.

Darling, Elizabeth. *Reforming Britain: Narratives of Modernity before Reconstruction*. London: Routledge, 2006.

Daston, Lorraine, and Elizabeth Lunbeck. "Introduction. Observation Observed." In *Histories of Scientific Observation*, edited by Lorraine Daston and Elizabeth Lunbeck, 1–9. Chicago, Ill.: University of Chicago Press, 2011.

Digby, Anne. *Diversity and Division in Medicine. Health Care in South Africa from the 1800s*. Oxford: Lang, 2006.

Donaldson, Frances. *Child of the Twenties*. London: Rupert Hart-Davis, 1959.

Dörre, Klaus, Stephan Lessenich and Hartmut Rosa. *Sociology, Capitalism, Critique*, London/New York: Verso, 2015.

Duncan, D.F. "The Peckham Experiment: A Pioneering Exploration of Wellness." *Health Values* 9(1985): 40–43.

Elkes, Joel. "Past/Future Conjoined: Note from the USA on the Present Edition." *Social Medicine* 4 (2009 [1985]): 192–194.

Elsas, M.J. "The Peckham Experiment: A Study of the Living Structure of Society." *Eugenics Review* 36, no. 1(1944): 31–32.

Etzemüller, Thomas. *Alva and Gunnar Myrdal: Social Engineering in the Modern World*. Lanham: Lexington Books, 2014.

Ewald, François. *L'état providence*. Paris: B. Grasset, 1986.

Fenton, Clive B. "PLAN. A Student Journal of Ambition and Anxiety." In *Man-Made Future: Planning, Education and Design in Mid-Twentieth-Century Britain*, edited by Ian Boyd Whyte, 174–190. London/New York: Routledge, 2007.

Finlayson, Geoffrey. *Citizen, State and Social Welfare in Britain 1830–1990*. Oxford: Clarendon Press, 1994.

Fleck, Ludwik. *Genesis and Development of a Scientific Fact*. Chicago: University of Chicago Press, 1981 [1935].

Fleming, C.M. "The Social Psychology of Education." *The Listener* (May 4, 1944).

Ford, Rosa. "The Peckham Health Centre. A Record of Pioneer Work in Building Up Positive Health." *Nursing Times* (February 2, 1948): 148–151.

Fraher, Amy L. *A History of Group Study and Psychodynamic Organizations*. London: Free Association Books, 2004.

Furedi, Frank. *Therapy Culture: Cultivating Vulnerability in an Uncertain Age*. London: Routledge, 2004.

Gazeley, Ian. *Poverty in Britain, 1900–1965*. Basingstoke/London: Palgrave Macmillan, 2003.

Gebhard, Bruno. "The Peckham Experiment." *Medical Care* 4(1944): 315–317.

Gilchrist, Ruth, and Tony Jeffs, eds. *Settlements, Social Change, and Community Action: Good Neighbours*. London/Philadelphia: Jessica Kingsley Publishers, 2001.

Gilson, Mary B. "Health a Family Problem." *Survey* (1931): 660.

Goldman, Marion S. *The American Soul Rush: Esalen and the Rise of Spiritual Privilege*. New York: New York University Press, 2012.

Goodway, David. "Anarchism and the welfare state: the Peckham Health Centre." *History & Policy* (May 1, 2007). Accessed www.historyandpolicy.org/papers/policy-paper-55.html (Accessed December 17, 2017).

Gowing, Mary. "Incentives to Parenthood. Some Data from the Pioneer Health Centre, Peckham." *Eugenics Review* 35, no. 2(1943): 39–41.

Griesecke, Birgit, et al. "Vorwort." In *Kulturgeschichte des Menschenversuchs im 20. Jahrhundert*, edited by Birgit Griesecke et al., 7–15. Frankfurt: Suhrkamp, 2009.

Gruffudd, Pyrs. "'Science and the Stuff of Life'. Modernist Health Centres in 1930s London." *Journal of Historical Geography* 27(2001): 395–416.

Hall, Lesley A. "The Archives of the Pioneer Health Centre, Peckham, in the Wellcome Library." *Social History of Medicine* 14(2001): 525–538.

Hardy, Anne. *Health and Medicine in Britain since 1860*. Basingstoke: Palgrave Macmillan, 2001.

Hardy, Dennis. *Utopian England. Community Experiments 1900–1945*. London: E & FN Spon, 2000.

Harrington, Anne. *Reenchanted Science. Holism in German Culture. From Wilhelm II to Hitler*. Princeton, NJ: Princeton University Press, 1996.

Harrison, Tom. *Bion, Rickman, Foulkes and the Northfield Experiments: Advancing on a Different Front*. London: Jessica Kingsley Publishers, 2000.

Hastings, Somerville. "Health Centres." *Comrade* (October 1946).

Haworth, Lawrence. *The Good City*. Bloomington: Indiana University Press, 1963.

Herbert, Ulrich. "Europe in High Modernity. Reflections on a Theory of the 20th Century." *Journal of Modern European History* 5, no. 1(2007): 5–21.

Hewetson, John. "Peckham Health Experiment." *Freedom* (1947).

Hewetson, John. "A Peckham Testament." *Anarchy* 6(1966): 61–64.

Hewitt, Jean F. "The Peckham Experiment." *The American Catholic Sociological Review* 7(1946): 139–140.

Hubble, Nick. *Mass Observation and Everyday Life. Culture, History, Theory*. Basingstoke: Palgrave Macmillan, 2006.

Humphreys, Robert. *Poor Relief and Charity 1869–1945. The London Charity Organization Society*. New York: Palgrave Macmillan, 2001.

Huxley, Aldous. *Brave New World Revisited*. New York: Harper & Brothers, 1958.

Huxley, Julian. *Scientific Research and Social Needs*. London: Watts & Co., 1934.

Huxley, Julian. *Memories*. Harmondsworth: Penguin Books, 1972.

Jackson, Ben. "The Origins of Neo-Liberalism: the Free Economy and the Strong State, 1930–1947." *The Historical Journal* 53(2010): 129–151.

Jackson, Mark. *The Age of Stress. Science and the Search for Stability*. Oxford: Oxford University Press, 2013.

Johnson, M.L. "Research in Social Organization. The Peckham Experiment." *Nature* 153(1944): 269–270.

Jones, Essylt. "Nothing Too Good for the People. Local Labour and London's Interwar Health Centre Movement." *Social History of Medicine* 25(2012): 84–102.

Jones, Greta. "Eugenics and Social Policy between the Wars." *Historical Journal* 25 (1982): 717–728.

Jones, Greta. *Social Hygiene in Twentieth Century Britain*. London: Croom Helm, 1986.

Joyce, Patrick. *Democratic Subjects. The Self and the Social in Nineteenth-Century England*. Cambridge/New York: Cambridge University Press, 1994.

King Hall, Stephen. "45 years ago – the Pioneer Health Centre, Peckham." *Journal of the Royal Society of Medicine* 82(1989): 577–578.

Kohn, Robert. *The Health Centre Concept in Primary Health Care*. [Geneva]: World Health Organization, 1983.

Koven, Seth. *Slumming, Sexual and Social Politics in Victorian London*. Princeton, NJ: Princeton University Press, 2004.

Kozlovsky, Roy. *The Architectures of Childhood. Children, Modern Architecture and Reconstruction in Postwar England*. London: Routledge, 2013.

Kuchenbuch, David. *Geordnete Gemeinschaft. Architekten als Sozialingenieure – Deutschland und Schweden im 20. Jahrhundert*. Bielefeld: Transcript, 2010.

Kühl, Stefan. *For the Betterment of the Race. The Rise and Fall of the International Movement for Eugenics and Racial Hygiene*. New York: Palgrave Macmillan, 2013.

Kuper, Leo. "Blueprint for Living Together." In *Living in Towns. Selected Research Papers in Urban Sociology of the Faculty of Commerce and Social Science University of Birmingham*, edited by Leo Kuper, 1–202. London: Cresset Press, 1953.

Lacan, Jacques. "English Psychiatry and the War." *Psychoanalytical Notebooks of the London Circle* 4(2000 [1947]): 9–34.

Lawrence, Christopher. "Regenerating England: An Introduction." In *Greater than the Parts: Holism in Biomedicine, 1920–1950*, edited by Christopher Lawrence and George Weisz, 1–23. Oxford: Oxford University Press, 1998a.

Lawrence, Christopher. "Still Incommunicable: Clinical Holists and Medical Knowledge in Interwar Britain" In *Greater than the Parts: Holism in Biomedicine, 1920–1950*, edited by Christopher Lawrence and George Weisz, 94–111. Oxford: Oxford University Press, 1998b.

Levene, Alysa. "Between Less Eligibility and the NHS: The Changing Place of the Poor Law Hospitals in England and Wales, 1929–1939." *Twentieth Century British History* 20(2009): 322–345.

Lewis, Jane, and Barbara Brookes. "A Reassessment of the Work of the Peckham Health Centre, 1926–1951." *Health and Society* 61(1983a): 307–350.

Lewis, Jane, and Barbara Brookes. "The Peckham Health Centre, 'PEP', and the Concept of General Practice during the 1930s and 1940s." *Medical History* 27 (1983b): 151–161.

Luckin, Bill. "Revisiting the Idea of Degeneration in Urban Britain, 1830–1900." *Urban History* 33(2006): 234–252.

Luckin, Bill, and Graham Mooney. "Urban History and Historical Epidemiology: The Case of London, 1860–1920." *Urban History* 24(1997): 37–55.

Luks, Timo. "The Factory as Environment. Social Engineering and the Ecology of Industrial Workplaces in Inter-War Germany." *European Review of History: Revue europeenne d'histoire* 20(2013): 271–285.

Mackintosh, James. *The Nation's Health*. London: Pilot Press, 1944.

Mawson, Andrew. *The Social Entrepreneur. Making Communities Work*. London: Atlantic, 2008.

Mayo, Elton. "Foreword," In *Management and the Worker. Technical vs. Social Organization in an Industrial Plant*, edited by Fritz Jules Roethlisberger and William J. Dickson, iii–vi. Cambridge, Mass.: Harvard University Press, 1934.

Mazumdar, Pauline M. *Eugenics, Human Genetics, and Human Failings: the Eugenics Society, its Sources and its Critics in Britain*. London: Routledge, 1992.

McGregor, Robert M. "Living and Dying." *British Medical Journal* (January 29, 1966): 238.

Metz, Karl H. "'Selbsthilfe'. Anmerkungen zu einer viktorianischen Idee." In *"Victorian Values". Arm und Reich im Viktorianischen England*, edited by Bernd Weisbrod, 98–125. Bochum: Brockmeyer, 1987.

Ministry of Health. Consultative Council on Medical and Allied Services. *Interim Report on the Future Provision of Medical and Allied Services 1920*. London: His Majesty's Stationery Office, 1920.

Ministry of Health. Department of Health for Scotland. *A National Health Service. Presented by the Minister of Health and the Secretary of State for Scotland to Parliament by Command of His Majesty*. London: Ministry of Health, 1944.

Moholy-Nagy, László. *Vision in Motion*. Chicago: Paul Theobald & Co., 1947.

Mold, Alex. "Making the Patient-Consumer in Margaret Thatcher's Britain." *The Historical Journal* 54(2011): 509–528.

Morgan, Arthur E. "Elements of Community Life." *Community Service News* 2, no. 3 (1944): 1–4.

Morgan, David, and Mary Evans. *The Battle for Britain. Citizenship and Ideology in the Second World War*. London/New York: Routledge, 1993.

The Museum of Modern Art. *Modern Architecture in England. With essays by Henry-Russell Hitchcock and Catherine K. Bauer*. New York: Museum of Modern Art, 1937.

Myrdal, Alva. "Hälsan är fritidsnöje i PECKHAM." *Vi* 33, no. 34(1946): 7–8.

n.a. "The Case for Action." *Review of Biology* 1, no. 1(1932): 16.

n.a. "Pioneer Health Centre, Peckham." *The Architectural Review* 77(1935): 209–216.

n.a. "VI. Internationaler Kongress für physikalische Therapie in London." *Deutsche Medizinische Wochenschrift* 29(1936a): 82.

n.a. "The Basis of Planning. A Lecture given at the School of Planning and Research for National Development by Dr. Scott Williamson." *Architectural Association Journal* (November 1936b): 182–186.

n.a. "Biological Aspects of Health. Biologists in Search of Material." *Nature* 142 (1938a): 134–135.

n.a. "Biologists in Search of Material." *Industrial Welfare* (1938b): 167.

n.a. "Biologists in Search of Material." *British Medical Journal* (1938c): 1312.

n.a. "The Peckham Health Centre. A Three-Years Survey." *British Medical Journal* (June 11, 1938d): 1056–1057.

n.a. "Peckham Health Centre." *Medical Officer* (July 1940).

n.a. "Centre of Public Health. First Steps in a Practical Plan." *Libertas* (December1943): 22–28.

n.a. *Planning. A Broadsheet issued by PEP*. [London], 1944a.

n.a. "The Peckham Experiment." *The Medical Officer* (January 1944b).

n.a. "A Revolutionary Scheme of Local Government." *British Medical Journal* (June 30, 1945a): 911–912.

n.a. "Excursion into Utopia." *Medical Press* (September 9, 1945b).

n.a. "Family Health." *The Lancet* (March 3, 1946): 355.

n.a. "George Scott Williamson." *The Lancet* (June 13, 1953): 1206–1207.

n.a. "The Nature of Health." *The Expository Times* (August 1966): 335.

n.a. *The Community Health Centre in Canada. Report of the Community Health Centre Project to the Health Ministers*. Ottawa: Information Canada, 1972/73.

n.a. *The Role of Health Centres in the Development of Urban Health Systems. Report of a WHO Study Group on primary Health Care in Urban Areas.* Geneva: World Health Organization, 1992.

O'Hara, Glen. "The Complexities of 'Consumerism': Choice, Collectivism and Participation within Britain's National Health Service, c. 1961–c. 1979." *Social History of Medicine* 25(2013): 288–304.

Palmer, Mary B. "Experiment in Health." *Harper's Magazine* (May 1949): 327–432.

Pearse, Innes H. "Racial Culture." *Journal of State Medicine* 44, no. 10(1927): 1–69.

Pearse, Innes H. "Positive Health." *British Medical Journal* (July 18, 1942): 78–79.

Pearse, Innes H. "What is a Health Centre?" *Public Health* (November 1944): 15–18.

Pearse, Innes H. "The Peckham Experiment." *Eugenics Review* 37, no. 2(1945): 48–55.

Pearse, Innes H. *The Quality of Life: The Peckham Approach to Human Ethology.* Edinburgh: Scottish Academic Press, 1979.

Pearse, Innes H., and Lucy H. Crocker. *The Peckham Experiment. A Study of the Living Structure of Society.* London: Allen & Unwin, 1943.

Pearse, Innes H., and George Scott Williamson. *Science, Synthesis and Sanity. An Enquiry into the Nature of Living.* London: Collins, 1965.

Pearson, Monica. "The Peckham Experiment: A Pioneer British Health Center." *The Social Service Review* 21(1947): 132–134.

Pemberton, John. "The Peckham-Experiment." *Journal of Public Health Policy* 12 (1991): 542–544.

Perkin, Harold. *The Rise of Professional Society. England since 1880.* London: Routledge, 1989.

Perls, Frederick S., Ralph Hefferline, and Paul Goodman. *Gestalt-Therapy. Excitement and Growth in the Human Personality.* New York: Dell, 1951.

Pethes, Nicolas. "Einleitung." In: *Menschenversuche. Eine Anthologie 1750–2000*, edited by Nicolas Pethes, 715–725, Frankfurt: Suhrkamp, 2008.

Pines, Malcolm, ed. *Bion and Group Therapy.* London: Jessica Kingsley Publishers, 2000.

Pines, Malcolm. "Large Groups and Culture." In *The large group re-visited: The herd, primal horde, crowds and masses*, edited by Stanley Schneider et al., 44–57. London: Jessica Kingsley Publishers, 2003.

Porter, Dorothy. *Health, Civilisation and the State. A History of Public Health from Ancient to Modern Times.* London: Routledge, 1992.

Porter, Dorothy. "Social Medicine and the New Society: Medicine and Scientific Humanism in mid-Twentieth Century Britain." *Journal of Historical Sociology* 9 (1996): 168–187.

Porter, Dorothy. "The decline of social medicine in Britain in the 1960s" In *Social medicine and medical sociology in the twentieth century*, edited by Dorothy Porter, 97–119. Amsterdam: Rodopi, 1997.

Rabinbach, Anson. *The Human Motor. Energy, Fatigue, and the Origins of Modernity.* Berkeley: University of California Press, 1992.

Ransom, Donald C. "Random Notes: The Legacy of the Peckham Experiment." *Family Systems Medicine* 10(1983): 104–108.

Raphael, Lutz. "Embedding the Human and Social Sciences in Western Societies, 1880–1980." In *Engineering Society. The Role of the Human and Social Sciences in Modern Societies 1880–1980*, edited by Kerstin Brückweh et al., 41–58. Basingstoke: Palgrave Macmillan, 2012.

Read, Herbert. "The Peckham Experiment." *The Listener* (December 23, 1943): 729.

Reed, Mathew. *Rebels for the Soil: The Rise of the Global Organic Food and Farming Movement*. London: Earthscan, 2010.

Renwick, Chris. *British Sociology's Lost Biological Roots: A History of Futures Past*. Basingstoke: Palgrave Macmillan, 2012.

Renwick, Chris. "Eugenics, Population Research, and Social Mobility Studies in Early and Mid-Twentieth-Century Britain." *The Historical Journal* 59(2016): 845–867.

Rheinberger, Hans-Jörg, and Michael Hagner. "Experimentalsysteme." In *Die Experimentalisierung des Lebens. Experimentalsysteme in den biologischen Wissenschaften 1850/1950*, edited by Hans-Jörg Rheinberger and Michael Hagner, 7–27. Berlin: Akademie Verlag, 1993.

Richards, J.M. "The Idea Behind the Idea." *The Architectural Review* 77(1935a): 207–209.

Richards, J.M. "Pioneer Work at Peckham." *The Architect's Journal* 81(1935b): 509.

Richards, J.M. "Finsbury Makes a Programme." *The Architectural Review* 85(1939): 9.

Richards, J.M. *Memoirs of an Unjust Fella*. London: Weidenfeld and Nicolson, 1980.

Ritschel, Daniel. *The Politics of Planning. The Debate on Economic Planning in Britain in the 1930s*. Oxford: Clarendon, 1997.

Roemer, Milton I. *Evaluation of Community Health Centres*. Geneva: World Health Organization, 1972.

Rogers, Maria. "The Peckham Experiment." *Sociometry* 8(1945): 92–96.

Rose, Nikolas. *Governing the Soul. The Shaping of the Private Self*. London: Routledge, 1990.

Rose, Nikolas. *Powers of Freedom: Reframing political thought*. Cambridge: Cambridge University Press, 1999.

Rose, Nikolas, and Peter Miller. "The Tavistock Programme: The Government of Subjectivity and Social Life." *Sociology* 22(1988): 171–192.

Ryle, J.A. "The Peckham Experiment." *Bulletin of Hygiene* (1944): 236.

Sargent Wood, Linda. *A More Perfect Union. Holistic Worldviews and the Transformation of American Culture after World War II*. New York/Oxford: Oxford University Press, 2010.

Savage, Mike. *Identities and Social Change in Britain since 1940. The Politics of Method*. Oxford: Oxford University Press, 2010.

Schildein Grimes, Sharon. *The British National Health Service. State Intervention in the Medical Marketplace, 1911–1948*. London: Routledge, 1991.

Scotland, Nigel. *Squires in the Slums: Settlements and Missions in Late-Victorian London*. London/New York: I.B. Tauris, 2007.

Scott, James C. *Seeing Like a State: How Certain Schemes to Improve the Human Condition Have Failed*. New Haven, Conn./London: Yale University Press, 1998.

Scott-Samuel, Axel. *Total Participation, Total Health: Reinventing the Peckham Health Centre for the 1990s*. Edinburgh: Scottish Academic Press, 1990.

Scott Williamson, George. *Physician, heal thyself: A Study of Needs and Means*. London: Faber & Faber, 1945.

Scott Williamson, George. "What is Science?" *Mother Earth* 6, no. 4(1952): 39–44.

Scott Williamson, George. "The Individual and the Community." In *The Heart of the City: Towards the Humanisation of Urban Life. CIAM 8/International Congresses for Modern Architecture*, edited by Jacqueline Tyrwhitt, José Luis Sert and Ernesto Rogers, 30–35. Nendeln: Kraus Reprint, 1979 [1952].

Scott Williamson, George, and Innes H. Pearse. "Evidence Drawn from a Study of the Therapeutics of Graves' Disease, of Two Functions in the Thyroid Physiology." *Quarterly Journal of Medicine* 22(1928): 21–31.

Scott Williamson, George, and Innes H. Pearse. *The Case for Action. A Survey of Everyday Life under Modern Industrial Conditions, with Special Reference to the Question of Health*. London: Faber & Faber, 1931.

Scott Williamson, George, and Innes H. Pearse. *Biologists in Search of Material. An Interim Report on the Work of the Pioneer Health Centre, Peckham*. London: Faber & Faber, 1938.

Shapira, Michal. *The War Inside: Psychoanalysis, Total War, and the Making of the Democratic Self in Postwar Britain*. Cambridge: Cambridge University Press, 2015.

Smith, Roger. "Biology and Values in Interwar Britain: C. S. Sherrington, Julian Huxley and the Vision of Progress." *Past & Present* 178(2003): 210–242.

Sommer, Marianne. "Die Biologie der Demokratie im Wissenschaftlichen Humanismus." In *Wissenschaft und Demokratie*, edited by Michael Hagner, 51–68. Frankfurt: Suhrkamp, 2012.

Stallibrass, Alison. *The Self-Respecting Child*. London: Thames and Hudson, 1974.

Stallibrass, Alison. *Being Me and Also Us. Lessons from the Peckham Experiment*. Edinburgh: Scottish Academic Press, 1989.

Stark Murray, David. "Doctors into Biologists." *Socialist Medical Association Bulletin* (September1947): 57.

Starkey, Pat. "The Medical Officer of Health, the Social Worker, and the Problem Family, 1943 to 1968: The Case of Family Service Units." *Social History of Medicine* 11(1998): 421–441.

Stewart, John. "'For a Healthy London': The Socialist Medical Association and the London County Council in the 1930s." *Medical History* 42(1997): 417–443.

Stewart, John. *"The Battle for Health." A Political History of the Socialist Medical Association, 1930–51*. Aldershot: Ashgate, 1999

Stewart, John. "The Political Economy of the British National Health Service, 1945–1975: Opportunities and Constraints?" *Medical History* 52(2008): 453–470.

Sturdy, Steve. "Hippocrates and the State Medicine: George Newman Outlines the Founding Policy of the Ministry of Health." In *Greater than the Parts: Holism in Biomedicine, 1920–1950*, edited by Christopher Lawrence and George Weisz, 112–134. Oxford: Oxford University Press, 1998.

Summer, G. "Plywood Furniture at the Pioneer Health Centre." *Design for Today* 3 (1935): 219–220.

Sutcliffe-Braithwaite, Florence. "Neo-Liberalism and Morality in the Making of Thatcherite Social Policy." *The Historical Journal* 55(2012): 497–520.

Tanner, Jakob. "'Weisheit des Körpers' und soziale Homöostase. Physiologie und das Konzept der Selbstregulation." In *Physiologie und industrielle Gesellschaft. Studien zur Verwissenschaftlichung des Körpers im 19. und 20. Jahrhundert*, edited by Jakob Tanner and Philipp Sarasin, 129–169. Frankfurt: Suhrkamp, 1998.

Thane, Pat. "The 'Big Society' and the 'Big State': Creative Tension or Crowding Out?" *Twentieth Century British History* 23(2012): 408–429.

Thomson, Mathew. *Psychological Subjects. Identity, Culture, and Health in Twentieth Century Britain*. Oxford: Oxford University Press, 2006.

Tomlinson, Jim. "Thrice Denied: 'Declinism' as a Recurrent Theme in British History in the Long Twentieth Century." *Twentieth Century British History* 20(2009): 227–251.

Trotter, J. Douglas. *Wholeness and Holiness. A Study in Human Ethology and the Holy Trinity*. Glasgow: Pioneer Health Foundation, 2003.

Turda, Marius. *Modernism and Eugenics*. Basingstoke: Palgrave Macmillan, 2010.

Tyrwhitt, Jacqueline. "Introduction." In *Cities in Evolution*, edited by Patrick Geddes, ix–xxviii. London: Williams and Norgate, 1949.

Walter-Busch, Emil. *Das Auge der Firma. Mayos Hawthorne-Experimente und die Harvard Business School, 1900–1960*. Stuttgart: F. Enke, 1989.

Ward, Colin. "Peckham Recollected." *Anarchy* 6(1966a): 52–56.

Ward, Colin. "'A Laboratory of Anarchy'. A Comparative Anthology." *Anarchy* 6 (1966b): 56–61.

Ward, Colin. "The organization of anarchy." In *Patterns of Anarchy. A Collection of Writings on the Anarchist Tradition*, edited by Leonard I. Krimerman and Lewis Perry, 349–351. New York: Anchor Books, 1966c.

Ward, Colin. "Fringe benefit." *New Statesman & Society* 213, no. 5(1992): 26.

Webb, Sidney, and Beatrice Webb, ed. *The Minority Report of the Poor Law Commission Part I: The Break-Up of the Poor Law*. Clifton: A.M. Kelley, 1979 [1909].

Webster, Charles. *The National Health Service: A Political History*. Oxford: Oxford University Press, 1998.

Werskey, Gary. *The Visible College. A Collective Biography of British Scientists and Socialists of the 1930s*. London: Free Association, 1988.

White, Kerr Lachlan. "Recent Contributions to the Science of Health." *McGill Medical Journal* (October 1947): 359–381.

Wills, David W. *The Hawkspur Experiment. An Informal Account of the Training of Wayward Adolescents*. London: Allen and Unwin, 1941.

Winner, I.H. "The End of the Peckham Experiment?" *Scientific Worker* 5, no. 4(1950): 18–21.

Young, Michael. "The Peckham Experiment." *Self Health* 10(1984): 11.

Zweiniger-Bargielowska, Ina. *Managing the Body. Beauty, Health, and Fitness in Britain 1880–1939*. Oxford: Oxford University Press, 2010.

Archives

BAB – *Bauhaus Archiv Berlin*
Papers of Walter Gropius

BPS – *Archives of the British Psychoanalytical Society*
P03/B/B/03 Rickman Papers

gta – *Archiv des Instituts für Geschichte und Theorie der Architektur an der ETH Zürich*

Jaqueline Tyrwhitt, 42-JT
Sigfried Giedion, 42-SG

LMA – *London Metropolitan Archives*
LCC, Public Health Department: Personal Health Services
LCC, Clerk's Department: Committees concerned with Public Health
GLC – Greater London Council

LSE – *London School of Economics and Political Science Archives*

COLL MISC 0521 Vernon; Wilfred Foulston (1882–1974); politician
WG 15 PEP Health Group

RIBA – *RIBA Study Room at the V&A, London*

Greh – Harry Stuart Goodhart-Rendel
Design for the Pioneer Health Centre, Saint Mary's Road, Peckham, Williams, Sir Evan Owen, 1890–1969, DR52/7
London (Southwark): Pioneer Health Centre, Camberwell, competition design, finished perspective, 1930, Musman, Ernest Brander, RAN 15/B/20(1)
London (Southwark): Pioneer Health Centre, Saint Mary's Road, Peckham, competition designs, ca. 1930, PA354/9(1–20)

Designs & working drawings for offices, cubicles, kitchen & furniture for the Pioneer Health Centre, Saint Mary's Road, Southwark, London by Christopher Nicholson. PA1206/4(1–58)

SLHA – *Southwark Local History Archives, London*

P 613 Health Centres
PC 613 Peckham Health Centre
PC 613 Photos
Tape 18: Mary Boast interviews Dr Innes Pearse, 23.6.1976

TNA – *The National Archives, Kew*

AVIA Records created or inherited by the Ministry of Aviation and successors, the Air Registration Board, and related bodies
MH Records created or inherited by the Ministry of Health and successors, Local Government Boards and related bodies
FD Records created or inherited by the Medical Research Council
ED Records created or inherited by the Department of Education and Science, and of related bodies

WL – *Wellcome Library for the History and Understanding of Medicine, London*

SA/PHC Pioneer Health Centre Peckham, with papers of George Scott Williamson MD (1884–1953) and Innes Hope Pearse (1889–1978)

Index

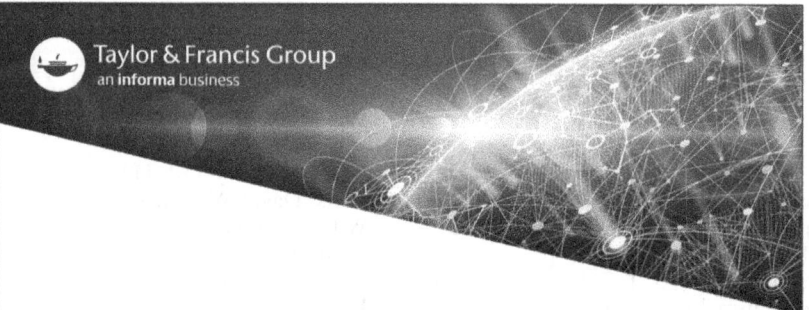
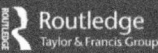
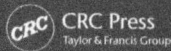